GET TO KNOW YOURSELF

GET TO KNOW YOURSELF

A training package for health promoters, health educators, community health workers and peer educators promoting sexual health among young people

THELMAH XAVELA MALULEKE

authorHOUSE®

AuthorHouse™ UK
1663 Liberty Drive
Bloomington, IN 47403 USA
www.authorhouse.co.uk
Phone: 0800.197.4150

Published by AuthorHouse 11/05/2014

ISBN: 978-1-4969-8565-1 (sc)
ISBN: 978-1-4969-8566-8 (hc)
ISBN: 978-1-4969-8567-5 (e)

CONTENTS

PART TWO

Get to know yourself: A handbook for health promoters and peer
educators facilitating sexual health among young people

INTRODUCTION
TO THE TRAINING PACKAGE

In many countries particularly developing, young people face different challenges related to their sexuality: environment, age, gender, poverty, unemployment, diseases which have an influence on their perception of the world, and themselves. Lack of information and guidance about sex and sexuality make young people vulnerable to physical, emotional and economic exploitation. In many societies the family and community traditionally provided youth with information and guidance about sex and sexuality as part of their initiation into adulthood. However, societal changes, for example poverty, rapid urbanisation, migration, education and religion, have destabilised this traditional way of sharing information and knowledge in many families and communities. Many parents leave their families to seek work leaving their children with no guidance and support. The destabilisation of the family and traditional community networks have resulted in young people receiving conflicting messages about sexuality from siblings, peers and the mass media which are often not validated by a trusted adult.

Research has shown that access to reliable and accurate sexual health information during adolescence is a vital component in the development of a healthy sexual adult life. Importantly, positive sexual health outcomes usually occur within an environment that is supportive, and when facilitation of sexual health education integrates knowledge, motivation and skills that empower young people to make the right choices. Young people who have acquired knowledge and skills in sexual health are able to make decisions about whether to be sexually active, enjoying sex based on mutual respect and understanding, and avoid the risk of sexually transmitted infections (STIs) and unplanned pregnancy. Sexual health education programmes have been introduced in schools as part of life orientation or life skills, health promotion and health education in many countries. Within the health services sexual health education has become an important component of health promotion programs and youth health services.

Sexual health education workshops promote positive sexual health and responsible sexual behaviour that minimises the incidence of sexually transmitted infections (STIs) and unplanned pregnancy. It reduces incidence and impacts of STIs and stigma and discrimination against HIV positive people. It increases awareness of information promoting sexual health and wellbeing. The Get to know yourself sexual health workshops in the "Get to know yourself: A training package for health promoters, health educators, community health workers and peer educators promoting sexual health among young people" package will assist in developing and facilitating sexual health workshops. The workshops will equip young people with current and factual information that will enable them to make healthy sexual choices and prevent un-intended pregnancies, exposure to sexually transmitted infections and sexual exploitation. The workshops are planned to: build young people's self esteem and confidence in individuals; assist young people in developing positive relationships with others; provide a safe environment in which young people will feel free to discuss related topics; promote individual responsibility for well-being; enable young people to make responsible choices and to deal more effectively with the challenges they may encounter throughout their lives.

The "Get to know yourself: A training package for health promoters, health educators, community health workers and peer educators promoting sexual health among young people" consists of two parts, Part one is a book entitled "Get to know yourself: A sexual health guide for young people" and Part Two a handbook entitled "Get to know yourself: A handbook for health promoters, health educators, community health workers and peer educators facilitating sexual health programmes among young people". The package was developed to assist under resourced communities and countries in accessing sexual health information that will have a positive impact on the lives of young people. This training package can also be used by health professionals and other professionals to facilitate sexual health workshops in schools, youth organisations or clubs and religious organisations.

PART ONE

Get to know yourself: A sexual health guide for young people

Thelmah Xavela Maluleke

ACRONYMS

HIV: Human Immunodefiency Virus
AIDS: Acquired Immune-Defiency Syndrome
STD: Sexually Transmitted Disease
STI: Sexually Transmitted Infection

INTRODUCTION

Welcome to "Get to know yourself: A sexual health guide for young people" where you are about to learn about the human body, puberty, relationships, sexually transmitted diseases and Human Immunodeficiency Virus (HIV) and Acquired Immune-Deficiency Syndrome (AIDS). You might have experienced, or are at present experiencing some developmental changes in your life, which might have left you with some unanswered questions. This book is intended to assist in answering some of your questions.

This book is meant for young people, aged 15 years and older, females and males, virgins and those who are already sexually active, who want to lead a healthy life. Young people are often faced with a huge responsibility of making decisions about their sexuality usually with little or no information, or with confusing information they obtain from their friends. This book gives information on sexual health that will enable you to feel confident about making decisions about your life. The book is easy to read, and makes it easy for young people whose parents find it challenging to talk to them about sexual health matters, to read it on their own.

"Get to know yourself: A sexual health guide for young people" aims at providing accurate information about sexual health that will enable young people to develop responsible sexuality, mutual respect between females and males, and good relationships that will result in the improvement of their quality of life. The book is meant to directly address the reader. The book came into existence as a result of my work as a researcher and lecturer in youth health, health promotion and public health that indicated limitations in accessing sexual health information among young people especially in under resourced areas of South Africa. To ensure book's relevance to the targeted youth, the topics covered in the book were suggested by women and girls during a study of puberty rites for girls, questions asked by students and young people who participated in sexual health workshops. Lastly, the limited access to sexual health information observed when working in under resourced communities and the alarming rates of HIV and AIDS in many under resourced communities in South Africa and other countries made me realise the need for an easy-to-read book that will be accessible to the majority of people – the youth in the stated age cohort.

The book will assist you in understanding yourself as a person and young people in general, the human body and gaining knowledge and skills that will enable you to:

- Form attitudes, beliefs and values about your body image, sexuality, development and interpersonal relationships;
- Take responsible steps to prevent teenage pregnancy, sexually transmitted infections (STI), HIV and AIDS.
- Ensure access to the sexual health information by all young people, the book could be translated into different languages as the need arise.

What is sexual health?

Sexual health is defined as the integration of physical, emotional, intellectual and social aspects of sexual being in ways that are positively enriching, and that enhance personality, communication and love. It is the ability to have an informed, enjoyable, and safe sex life, based on a positive approach to sexual expression and mutual respect in sexual relations. In other words, sexual health means freedom from diseases, good relationship with yourself and others, and access to information that can enhance sexuality and relationships.

Sexual health acknowledges that human beings are sexual beings and have sexual rights. As sexual beings young people need to express and enjoy their sexuality throughout life and to take responsibility for their sexual behaviour. For you to exercise your sexual rights you need information, education, skills, support and services to make responsible decisions about your sexuality consistent with your own values. You need freedom from fear, shame, guilt, false beliefs and other factors that might inhibit your sexual response and impair your sexual relationship. As a sexually healthy person you appreciate your body, take responsibility for your behaviour, and communicate with people in a respectful manner. You probably communicate respectfully with both females and males, young and old.

You also communicate effectively with family, peers and partners. You seek information to make informed choices, express love and intimacy consistent with your values in an appropriate way and you protect yourself from unwanted pregnancy, STIs and HIV/AIDS. In other words, a sexually healthy individual makes informed choices and does not engage in a sexual relationship that will later embarrass her or him. As a sexually healthy person you know your rights and you respect those of others. You are able to have a relationship that is non-exploitative and is based on shared values, honesty, and mutual pleasure.

This book is based on the premise that a person is a physical being (biological composition), emotional being (self-concept), social being (relationships) and sexual being and that sexual health is the integration of the physical, emotional and social aspects of the person's sexual being. Your emotional being can affect your physical being, social being and sexual being. The same is true of your social being: it can affect how you see yourself, feel about yourself and your sexual behaviour. What is good about this relationship is that if you improve your emotional being (self-concept) you can improve all the others. In other words, building your self-concept is the key to improving your wellbeing, including sexual health. Since the self-concept is the main key to our lives, our discussion will start with the emotional being and progress to the physical being and lastly the social being.

This book is based on the premise that a person is a physical being (biological composition), emotional being (self-concept), social being (relationships) and sexual being and that sexual health is the integration of the physical, emotional and social aspects of the person's sexual being. As a result of the multi-dimensional composition of our 'being', this book is divided into five chapters. **Chapter 1:** "Who am I" introduces young people to the emotional or psychological component of their being, i.e. the self-concept and emotions. **Chapter 2:** "What does my body look like?" introduces youth to the physical being, which is the human body, its functions and human development. **Chapter 3** discusses the social component, which includes relationships with self, family, friends and partner. **Chapter 4** discusses how young people can keep themselves healthy. This chapter combines all three aspects of a human being. **Chapter 5** discusses virginity and issues related to it. **Chapter 6** discusses issues and consequences of being sexually active including contraception. **Chapter 7** discusses sexually transmitted infections (STI), HIV and AIDS and cancers affecting the reproductive system. **Chapter 8** discusses gender issues in sexual health. To clarify some of the issues, activities, stories and poems are used in some of the chapters.

CHAPTER 1

WHO AM I?

Exercise 1: What my name means.

Take a few minutes and do the following exercise. Write down your name and its meaning (if you know what it means). Who gave you the name? What is your relationship with the person who gave you your name? Are you named after someone? What does your name mean to you?

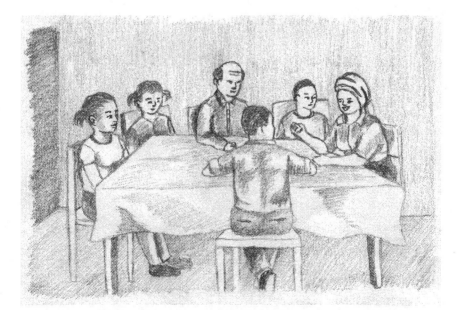

In many South African cultures a child is given a name immediately after birth or within a few days of its birth. Names can also be given at different stages of a person's life for example, in some cultures where initiation is practised, a person is given a new name during initiation and in some cultures you are given a new name when you are married. It is also common among teenagers, especially boys, to give themselves new names that are used by their friends and peers, or used during sporting activities. Whatever the circumstances may be, your name is very important to you as an individual. A name is the first thing that identifies a person as an individual. You could share a name with an individual or even be named after a particular person, but you do not become that person. You remain yourself. You cannot be that person and that person cannot be you. You are a unique human being who is special and different from other people in many ways. You will not find a person who is your duplicate anywhere in the whole world. There are many factors that define who you are. For example, size, height, nationality, sex, colour, your accomplishment, etc. These factors give us the sense of being individual.

The question "Who am I?" requires an individual to identify her/himself from other people. It requires you to define yourself as you see yourself (self-awareness). In your mind, as a human being you form a picture of who you are. In other words, you form an image of your self-identity. The image that you form about yourself influences your view about your appearance, performance and relationships. This image that you form about yourself is called your self-concept. Self-concept is based on what has happened to you throughout your life. It is formed by what people say to you, what you believe people say about you, how they look at you, what you achieve, i.e. your positive or negative achievements. The support and encouragement you get from your parents, family, peers and teachers also have a great influence on the development of your self-concept. Self-concept reveals your emotional maturity, and gives feelings of being wanted, accepted and cared for. It also gives you feelings of worth, adequacy, courage and ability to face life with all its challenges.

Many people struggle with their self-concept at one stage or another, for example during crisis situations. For young people this is more common during puberty, when they experience physical changes. The physical changes are part of a normal developmental stage. However, for young people who are not well prepared for the changes, these could become a crisis situation in their lives. If you have a positive self-concept you have probably accepted these changes and feel comfortable and satisfied with the way you are. You think positively and feel good about yourself and others. You feel good about your character and your qualities, and take pride in your abilities, skills and accomplishment. You probably do not do things that can hurt yourself or others and do not use put-downs or laugh at other people (Put-downs are humiliating or critical remarks). You do not discriminate against people because of their colour, location, sex or tribal origin. You treat them with respect and as equals. If you happened to hurt someone unintentionally, you apologise for your action and do not repeat your mistake.

Your good self-concept helps you to enjoy and do better at school. You tend to have better relationships with yourself, family, teachers, friends, peers and partner and feel happier. You also find it easier to deal with disappointments and failures. You do not blame others when you do not achieve your goals as planned, and you accept your mistakes. You realise that you are just human, and as a human being, you are capable of making mistakes at one stage or another. As a person with a good self-concept you have feelings of empathy and love towards other people. Your positive self-concept allows you to grow into a responsible adult with a healthy attitude towards life as a whole.

There are some young people however, who, because of their experiences and memories of the past, struggle and find it difficult to handle crisis situations and eventually develop a poor or lower self-concept. Poor self-concept also results from the negative things you say or what people say about you. Young people with a low self-concept usually have negative thoughts and feelings about themselves and their bodies. These negative thoughts and feelings make a person think poorly or negatively about her/himself and have put-down tendencies towards themselves. They often engage themselves in activities that could be harmful. For example, they may drink or do drugs to help themselves feel better.

When people lose their sense of self, they also lose their ability to empathise with other people. They feel rejected and frustrated, which makes them become hostile towards themselves and others. Hostility affects their sense of worthiness and makes them feel guilty and blame themselves and others for what is happening to them. The good news is that you can, as an individual, improve your self-concept and live a good life of success and happiness.

Remember 1.1: You might not like your name or its meaning, but remember, it is just a name. What is important is, **you**! You are a unique human being who is special and different from other people in many ways.

What can I do to develop or improve my self-concept?

To build your self-concept you need to develop skills to make you feel good about yourself. You have to strengthen your communication and assertive skills. You also need to develop those social skills that will enable you to negotiate throughout your life.

1. Feeling good about yourself.

Take a sheet of paper and draw a line that divides it into two equal parts. At the top of the left-hand side write "labels given to me" and write on the right-hand side, "What I am". Write down all the negative or bad labels given to you by yourself and others that you can remember. On the opposite side (what I am) write the opposite of each word or phrase you have written. The word or phrase must be positive. Try and remember all the positive things your family and other people have said about you and add them to the positive side. Write as many positive statements as possible. Begin your sentence with "I am". See the example below:

Negative labels given to me by myself or others	What I am.
E.g. I am unattractive.	e.g. I am beautiful

When you have finished writing, cut the paper along the dividing line and destroy the left side. You have now removed all the negative labels. Read the positive labels as many times as you possibly can. Duplicate it if you want to, and keep them in places where you will be able to read them. You can paste them next to a mirror or keep them in your purse or in your desk. Keep the paper in a place that is comfortable for you.

It is important to realise that the negative labels that are given to you by yourself and others prevent you from achieving success in whatever you are doing. These kinds of labels destroy your confidence and make you feel bad about yourself. These types of feelings can stop you from making friends or even performing well at school. It is important to rid yourself of these labels and the change starts with you. It is your responsibility and your right to love and believe in yourself and you can do it.

This is what you can do to claim back your self-concept:

- Think about yourself in a positive way.
- Always pay attention to the inner beauty in yourself and in others.
- Learn to make peace with yourself.
- Consciously pay attention to your thoughts.
- Ask yourself what you are you saying about yourself when you are alone.
- If you always catch yourself saying bad or negative things about yourself consciously take the thought out and replace it with a positive one.
- Avoid comparing yourself with other people. Comparing yourself with other people is very damaging to your self-concept.
- Make a habit of praising yourself every morning when you wake up, and appreciating the good day that is in front of you.
- Feel motivated to face the day and life in general.
- Feel in charge of what is happening to you and around you and feel confident to face the challenges of life.
- Always apply your energy to what you are doing and always do your best in order to achieve the best.
- Every night before you go to bed, write down at least two things about yourself that made you happy on that day.
- Participate in what is happening at home and in your community.
- Pay more attention to what you love, and do things you love.

- Avoid negative people or those who always say negative things to you and spend more time with people you care about.

- Avoid people who are always complaining and dissatisfied about everything that is happening in their lives or around them.

- Avoid noisy and domineering people, because they often use put-downs (put-downs are words or phrases that are used to make another person feel small or embarrassed).

- Develop a sense of humour, look at life in a positive way and enjoy it.

- Always walk with your chin up and appreciate your environment and the beautiful faces of the people you meet in the street.

- Take ownership of your life and strive for happiness by making decisions for yourself. You can do it!

- If you find that your self-concept is too much to handle on your own, consult a counsellor, psychologist or health provider. Yes, with good professional support you can do it!

2. Strengthening your communication skills

Communication and assertive skills are the next skills you need to improve your self-concept. Communication is very important in the interaction among people. Communication means sending messages to and receiving messages from someone else. Communication can be verbal (using words) and non-verbal (body language). When you communicate make sure that the message you send is clear so that the receiver will understand it the way you want her/him to understand it. Always speak clearly so that the person you are talking with will understand what you are saying. Pay attention to your non-verbal communication. Ensure that your body language supports what you are saying. For example, if you say "No", your body language should also show that you are saying "No" and that you mean it.

Another important communication skill you need is listening. Let the people you are talking with know you are listening by facing them when they talk to you. Stop doing whatever it was that you were busy with when they started speaking and look at them. Listen with warmth and respect for the other person. Check whether you have heard correctly. Avoid interruptions and allow them to say what they want to until everything has been said. Lastly, avoid finishing their sentences for them, because it gives the impression that you are in a hurry, and it can discourage the other persons from continuing with what they wanted to say.

3. Strengthening your assertive skills

There are three main ways in which you might respond when a situation arises in your life. These responses are assertive behaviour, non-assertive (unassertive) behaviour and aggressive behaviour. The following are responses from three boys who were asked to respond to the situation described below:

Exercise 2: Assertive skills

Imagine you are staying in an area where you need to fetch water from a communal tap, borehole or well. You come back from school tired, and find that there is no drinking water at home. Your brother is home and playing cards with his friends. How would you respond?

James: *I will say nothing, because I know that he is doing it purposely in order to hurt me.*

Langa: *I would say, you lazy idiot. How can you play cards when there is no water in this house? Do think I like fetching water for you every day?*

Larry: *I would say I am annoyed, because you almost always leave the fetching of water to me. I want us to work out a timetable so that we can share this responsibility.*

James's response is unassertive. When you are unassertive you are often hesitant, embarrassed and feel you are unimportant and your own needs will not be taken seriously. Non-assertive behaviour hurts your self-concept and makes you feel worthless and depressed. Non-assertive people's rights are often violated and this causes unnecessary stress. Non-assertive people do not say what they want. They usually beat about the bush and make other people guess what they want. By doing this they manipulate others so that they can get what they want without being honest and direct. Avoid unassertive behaviour and learn to be assertive.

Langa has been aggressive in his response. When you are aggressive you express your feelings and opinions in a threatening and pushy way. You often attack people and say what you want to say without regarding the feelings and rights of others. You try to get your way by dominating and overpowering others. Your behaviour threatens others and can even be violent towards others. Avoid aggressive behaviour and learn to be assertive.

Larry has responded assertively. Larry told his brother how he feels and also made a suggestion about the solution. When you are assertive you tell a person what you want, or need or would prefer. You state this clearly and confidently. You stand up for your rights, express honest feelings comfortably, preferences and opinions clearly. You exercise your personal right without denying the rights of other. As an assertive person you show respect for both yourself and others. You are in control of yourself and behave in ways that will make you feel good about yourself and others. It means developing a caring, honest and accepting relationship with others. As an assertive person you have the ability to ask for support when you need it. Assertive behaviour promotes equality in human relationships. It enables you to act in your own best interests, to stand up for yourself without anxiety. Assertive behaviour builds your self-confidence.

4. Have good social skills

Social skills are skills that enable an individual to be accepted in a society and to accept social norms that provide the foundation for adult social behaviour. To be accepted in the community you need to build positive relationships with your family, friends, teachers and the community. You need to develop negotiation skills that enable you to negotiate with self and others. **See chapter 2** for more discussion of social skills.

WHAT DOES MY BODY LOOK LIKE?

Exercise 3: Stomach pains

It is a Saturday afternoon. A group of teenagers is going to watch a soccer match at their local soccer field.

Patty: *Yoo! Puts her hand on her lower abdomen.*

Nono: *What is wrong Patty?*

Patty: *Hmm! I had this terrible stomach pain, but it is now gone.*

Molly: *Stomach pains! Where? Show me.* (Patty indicates where she had the pain). *Patty the stomach is not over there, you have intestines there. I think you just had some gas in your intestines.*

Paul: *How do you know all that?*

Molly: *I did human biology in my old school when I was in Grades 8 and 9. I enjoyed it. I also have a book with some pictures that show the different systems of the human body.*

Lucy: *You know Molly; I am so interested in knowing how my body functions, but unfortunately I also love my commercial subjects. I cannot take biology as one of my subjects you know.*

Molly: *I can teach you if you are interested.*

All of them: *Yaa! Molly, please teach us.*

Molly: *Yes, I will, but when?*

All of them: *Now! Molly.*

Lucy: *We have more than two hours before the match starts. Go and fetch your picture book.*

Molly: *I am back. The title of my book is "What does my body look like?"*

They all sat down and form a circle. For each system that she was talking about she showed them a picture.

Do you want to know how your body functions? Please join Molly and her friends in their lesson, "What does my body look like?" discussed below.

What does my body look like?

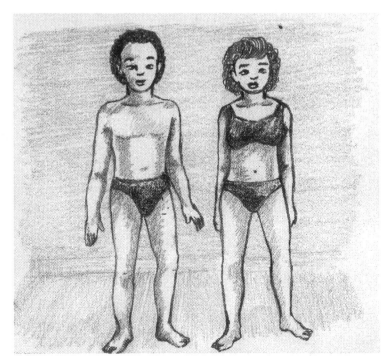

A diagram of the human body

The human body consists of different systems that work together to form a whole. The body functions like a machine, car or bicycle. The different parts should work together in order for it to function properly. The body functions in the same way. When you look at yourself you just see one person, but inside you there are ten systems working very hard to keep you alive. You do not hear or feel the systems working unless there is a problem.

The skin

When you look at yourself what you see is the skin. The skin covers the whole body. It consists of cells packed together, hair and nails. It protects the body from the sun, dust and germs. Germs are tiny organisms that cause diseases. They are so small that they can enter your body without your noticing. You need a microscope to see them. There are four types of germs: bacteria, viruses, fungi and protozoa.

The skin also helps to regulate the body temperature through sweating. Nails protect the sensitive tips of the fingers and toes. Hair grows everywhere on the body except on the palms of the hands, soles of the feet and the lips. The skin gets its colour from a pigment called melanin. Melanin protects the skin from the rays of the sun and prevents cancer of the skin. The more melanin you have the darker your skin is, and the less melanin you have, the fairer your skin is. Under the skin you find muscles.

Remember 2.1: Your skin colour does not make you superior or inferior to any person of a different colour.

The muscular system

This is the fleshy part of the body. It consists of different muscles that cover the bone structure, called the skeleton. The muscles join the different bones of the skeleton to form joints and enable them to move. They protect the bones and together with the bones they protect the internal organs of the body.

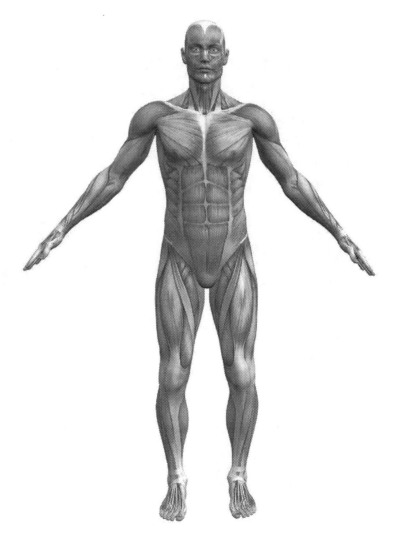

Graphics of muscles

The skeletal system

The skeletal system is the bony part of the body. It gives shape to the body and protects important organs of the body. For example, the ribs protect the heart and lungs and the skull protects the brain. In the bones there is bone marrow, which is also responsible for the manufacturing of blood cells.

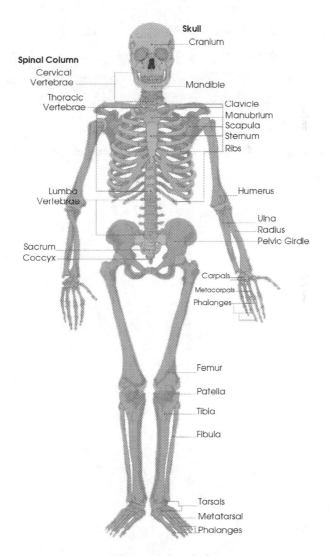

Skull
Cranium

Spinal Column
Cervical
Vertebrae

Mandible

Thoracic
Vertebrae

Clavicle
Manubrium
Scapula
Sternum
Ribs

Lumba
Vertebrae

Humerus

Ulna
Radius
Pelvic Girdle

Sacrum
Coccyx

Carpals
Metacarpals
Phalanges

Femur

Patella

Tibia

Fibula

Tarsals
Metatarsal
Phalanges

Graphics of the skeleton

The circulatory system

This system consists of the heart and a network of blood vessels called arteries and veins. The arteries further divide into smaller vessels that further divide and form tiny blood vessels called capillaries. The capillaries connect the arteries and veins in the tissues. The arteries transport blood from the heart to the different parts of the body while veins transport blood from all parts of the body to the heart. The blood that is carried by the arteries is often referred to as 'pure', because it contains nutrients and oxygen. Blood carried by the veins is often referred to as 'impure' blood because it carries carbon dioxide and waste products. The impure blood is purified by the respiratory and urinary system. The nutrients in the blood come from the digestive system. The blood carries all the nourishment that our bodies need, i.e. food, oxygen and hormones. Carbon dioxide is transported back to the lungs to be exhaled.

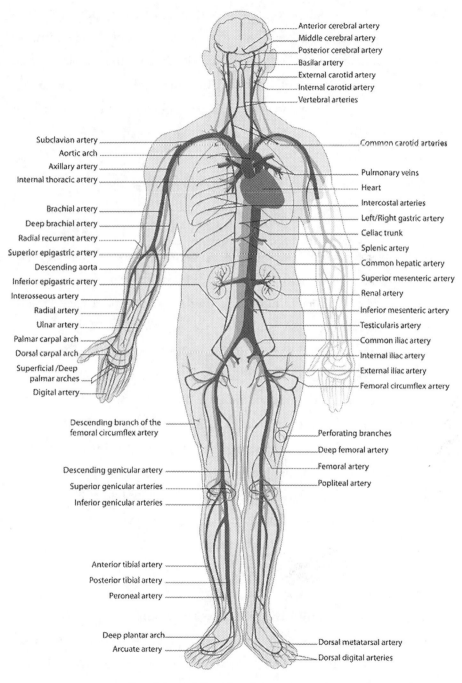

Anterior cerebral artery
Middle cerebral artery
Posterior cerebral artery
Basilar artery
External carotid artery
Internal carotid artery
Vertebral arteries

Subclavian artery
Aortic arch
Axillary artery
Internal thoracic artery

Common carotid arteries

Pulmonary veins
Heart
Intercostal arteries

Brachial artery
Deep brachial artery
Radial recurrent artery
Superior epigastric artery
Descending aorta
Inferior epigastric artery
Interosseous artery
Radial artery
Ulnar artery
Palmar carpal arch
Dorsal carpal arch
Superficial /Deep
palmar arches
Digital artery

Left/Right gastric artery
Celiac trunk
Splenic artery
Common hepatic artery
Superior mesenteric artery
Renal artery
Inferior mesenteric artery
Testicularis artery
Common iliac artery
Internal iliac artery
External iliac artery
Femoral circumflex artery

Descending branch of the
femoral circumflex artery

Perforating branches
Deep femoral artery

Descending genicular artery
Superior genicular arteries
Inferior genicular arteries

Femoral artery
Popliteal artery

Anterior tibial artery
Posterior tibial artery
Peroneal artery

Deep plantar arch
Arcuate artery

Dorsal metatarsal artery
Dorsal digital arteries

Graphics of the circulatory system

Blood consists of a high percentage of water called serum, mineral salts and blood cells. There are red and white blood cells and platelets in the blood. The platelets are responsible for blood clotting. The red blood cells carry oxygen to all parts of the body. The white cells protect the body from germs, i.e. bacteria and viruses. The white blood cells build up the immune system of the body. It is important to realise that there are millions of bacteria that attack the human body every second, but the skin, mucus membranes, acids in our body and white blood cells protect us from them.

White blood cells are in a continuous fight against bacteria and viruses. Most of the times they win the fight and you never even know you had some bacteria in your body. This means your body has good resistance and therefore, your immune system is functioning properly. Sometimes, in their quest to protect the body, the white blood cells get killed, but more are produced to keep the fight going. In the process of producing more cells the body gets tired, and then you start feeling ill and feverish. (Remember, the invaders are many and they keep on attacking and spitting toxic substances into your body and your body keeps on fighting and your illness becomes severe). In this case your body needs assistance, for example medicines that can kill the invading bacteria or virus. When your body can still fight strongly, your immune system is still working very well.

When your body is weak, some opportunistic germs get a chance of joining in the attack. When they multiply and your white blood cells (soldiers) are getting tired, the germs start attacking all systems in your body. Some of the germs the attack the lymph nodes and bone marrow and destroy them to stop them from producing white blood cells. When the invaders take over the lymph nodes and bone marrow, they destroy that person's immune system. Then the person is said to have a low resistance and immune deficiencies. Getting treatment and care can give your body the strength to start fighting back and eventually winning the battle against the germs.

Remember 2.2: You can minimise the attacks from bacteria by keeping yourself and your environment clean. Eat food that builds your body. Do not involve yourself in dangerous acts.

The lymphatic system

The lymphatic system consists of lymph nodes, lymph ducts and a network of lymphatic vessels. The lymph nodes are found throughout the body. Running through the vessels is a fluid called lymph. The lymphatic system flows from the body tissues toward the blood stream, returning fluid to the circulatory system. The lymph nodes are responsible for the formation of white blood cells. They also filter the lymph fluid that bathes the body tissues before it is emptied into the blood. The lymphatic system is also responsible for the protection of the body against germs. The lymphatic system is closely related to the circulatory system because it empties its lymph into the blood stream.

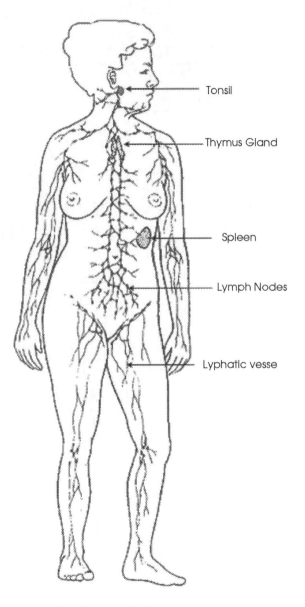

Graphics of the lymphatic system

The respiratory system

The respiratory system consists of the nose, trachea (air pipe), lungs and a network of bronchus, bronchioles and alveoli. The alveoli are responsible for the interchange of oxygen and carbon dioxide in the body. Capillaries surround the alveoli. When we breathe in, air-containing oxygen enters the lungs and passes to the alveoli. As the oxygen passes through the alveoli it is picked up by the red cells that pass through the alveoli. Oxygen is responsible for purifying the blood. It is carried to the heart and pumped out to the rest of the body.

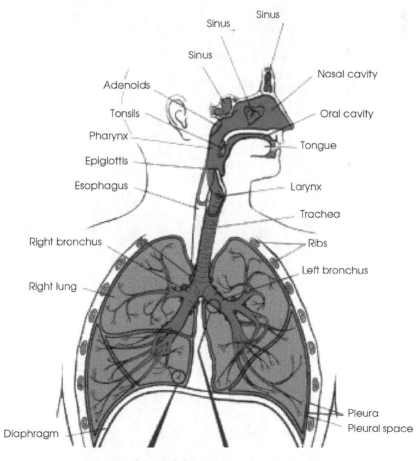

Graphics of the respiratory system

The digestive system

The digestive system consists of the mouth, oesophagus, stomach, intestines, rectum and anus. The liver, pancreas, gall bladder and the salivary glands form part of the digestive system. The digestive system breaks down and processes food and changes it into nutrients that dissolve into the blood and are carried to the different parts of the body. Food that cannot be used by the body is passed out through the rectum as waste products.

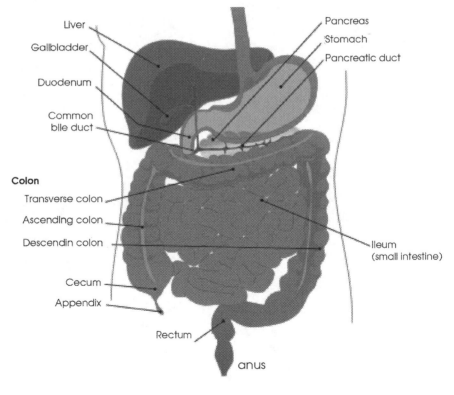

Graphics of the digestive system

The urinary system

The urinary system is the system that removes waste products from the blood. It consists of the kidneys, ureters, urinary bladder and urethra. The kidneys filter blood and produce urine. The kidneys also control blood pressure and the level of salts and other chemicals in the body. Excess salts, water and other waste products are removed from the body through urination.

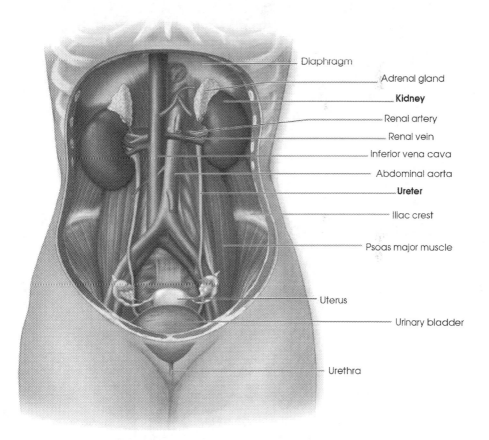

Graphics of the urinary system

The endocrine system

The endocrine system is the system that secretes hormones into the blood. The hormones are responsible for certain reactions in our body. For example, adrenaline helps us to run away from danger. The growth hormone helps us to grow. Oestrogen and progesterone stimulate the development of female secondary sexual characteristics and control of the menstrual cycle. Testosterone stimulates the development of male secondary sexual characteristics. It also supports the production of sperm by the testes.

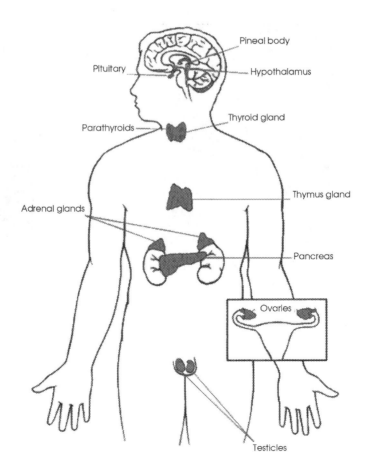

Graphics of the endocrine system

The nervous system

The nervous system consists of the brain, spinal cord and a network of nerves to and from the body. It is responsible for controlling the activities of the body by sending stimuli/messages to the different parts of the body. Because of the nervous system we can feel pain, hear, smell, see and walk.

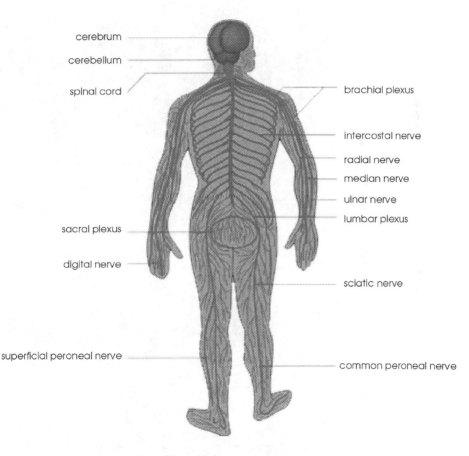

cerebrum
cerebellum
spinal cord
brachial plexus
intercostal nerve
radial nerve
median nerve
ulnar nerve
lumbar plexus
sacral plexus
digital nerve
sciatic nerve
superficial peroneal nerve
common peroneal nerve

Graphics of the nervous system

The reproductive system

The reproductive system is the system that is responsible for procreation and multiplication of people in the world. Females and males have different reproductive organs, often referred to as sex organs.

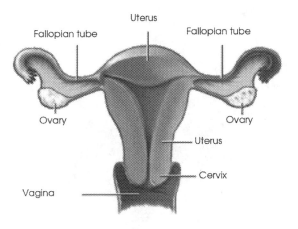

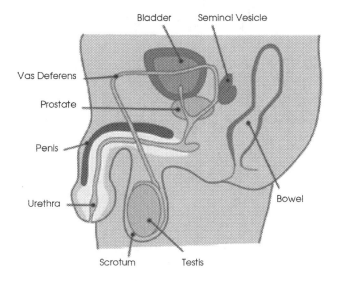

Graphics of male and female reproductive organs

I hope you have enjoyed the discussion with Molly. Take a few minutes and think about the questions below:

- Why is it important to understand the human body and how it functions?
- How are you going to use this information in your own life?
- What are you going to do to ensure that your friends also get the knowledge about their bodies that you have about yours?

> **Remember 2.3:** The difference in your reproductive organs or sex organs does not make you superior or inferior to a person of the opposite sex. They only define who you are and why your parents gave you the name you have. All that is important is to respect ourselves and each other and leave happily.

The human developmental stages

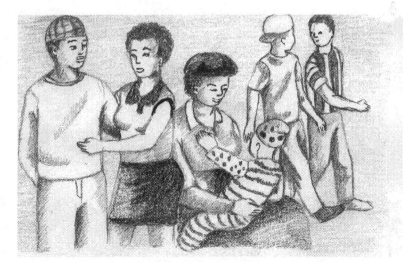

Exercise 4

Take some time to think about yourself when you were still a child and the different stages you have gone through until now. If you have some pictures of yourself at different stages of your development, paste them on a sheet of paper and compare them. What changes do you see? If you do not have pictures, just move on to the diagram below.

The diagrams above show the developmental stages of human beings, males and females. They illustrate the different stages and changes that occur from infancy to adulthood.

Infant

Childhood

Adolescence (puberty)

Adulthood

Developmental changes or signs of growth are noticeable from the day that you are born until you die. The signs of growing are changes in weight, height, emotions and how we relate to other people. As a human being we grow from infancy to childhood, and from childhood to adolescence, which is where the major changes happen in a person's life. The changes affect the way you look, feel, think and relate to others.

Adolescence (puberty)

Girls and boys reach the stage of puberty at different ages. Some people develop much earlier than their age groups whereas others develop much later than other people of the same age. During this stage you start to develop sexual feelings and interest in people of the opposite sex. Some young people start having relationships. The changes that happen during puberty are signs that you are becoming a responsible adult.

In order to grow into a responsible human being you need love, support and good relationships with your family. You need parents or guardians that love and guide you and at the same time you also need to love yourself and your parents or guardians. The development of appropriate and satisfying relationship with your family, friends and community depend upon your relationship with yourself. You cannot be well adjusted and happy if you have not accepted the normal developmental changes that are happening in your life. You cannot relate well to your family, friends and community if you are not happy with yourself. You cannot have a healthy sexual life if your personal relationship is not good. It is therefore important to build a good relationship with yourself and others.

Remember 2.4: Growing up means taking responsibility for your life. You cannot have a good relationship with your family, friends, partner and community if you do not love yourself.

Developmental changes in girls

Puberty in girls usually starts between the ages of 8 and 16 years. At this stage girls develop breasts, grow hair on the pubis and in the armpits. Their sexual organs become bigger and fuller. The hips become curvier and you grow taller. At a later stage their menstruation (menses or periods) starts.

Menstruation

A woman in a sexual health workshop told the story below. If the story sounds familiar, it is because you are not alone. Many young people experience this because of lack of information about their developmental stages.

The story of Margaret

When I got my first menses I was doing standard five. It came to me as a shock. I did not know that one day I would have menses. Just imagine sitting in class wearing a sky blue tunic and it happens. It was break time. As usual I rushed out of classroom and went straight to the playground. I think the first people who saw what has happened were two standard three boys. You know I cannot tell you what exactly happened there after, but I remember seeing them point at me saying she slept with boys. I remember looking over my shoulder and there was nobody behind me. A group of kids were running towards me pointing at the big red patch on my tunic. I got a shock of my life when I saw the blood. I was still puzzled when two of my classmates pushed through the crowd and tied a jersey on my waist and escorted me home. I was now crying bitterly, because I knew that I did not sleep with boys, but I could not understand where the blood came from. The two girls comforted me and told me I had my first menses and that it was normal. I stayed away from school for a week, in actual fact I was too embarrassed to go back to school.

Many girls learn about menstruation when they have had the menses themselves. They often have traumatic experiences, because of lack of knowledge about their normal development. They describe their experience as distressing, and full of apprehension and panic. Those who have knowledge perceive menstruation as a normal episode in their lives and have no fear or complaint about its onset.

As a girl you are born with hundreds of immature eggs in your ovaries. When you reach puberty the eggs start developing and maturing. Only one egg matures per month. The day you see your first menses is the commencement of a cycle of hormonal action that happen in your body in preparation for pregnancy. Most girls start menstruating between 11 and 16 years of age and continue with their periods until menopause. When a woman fails to have her periods before menopause it usually means she is pregnant or she has a serious condition that needs a doctor's attention.

Menstrual cycle

The menstruation cycle is about 28 days, but it differs according to individuals. Some have longer cycles while others have shorter. Remember, the female sex hormones oestrogen and progesterone discussed under the endocrine system. Every month oestrogen is sent to the ovaries to prepare the egg. At the same time it works on the inside of the uterus for a possible pregnancy. It causes the inner lining of the uterus to grow very fast, and blood vessels to swell and become engorged with blood. It makes a nice cushion for a fertilised egg if you happen to have had sexual intercourse, and a sperm has fertilised it. The fertilised egg will then attach itself to the cushion and start growing. This means that you are pregnant and there won't be menses from that time until you have the baby. If no fertilisation has taken place, the inside lining of the uterus crumbles and you have your menses. Menstruation or having a period happens when the lining of the girl's womb runs out of the vagina in the form of blood. It is not a sign of illness or dirtiness, but a normal sign that you are not pregnant. During menstruation you need to use sanitary pads or tampons. Many people who cannot afford these use toilet paper. Whatever you use, you need to change it regularly. Keep yourself clean. Wash yourself at least twice a day, in the morning and before going to bed.

Menstruation is often painless, but sometimes it is accompanied by stomach cramps or severe headaches or vomiting, which is called menstrual pains or dysmenorrhoea. If your menstrual pains are unbearable or interfere with your normal activities, visit your clinic or doctor.

> **Remember 2.5:** Having sex during menstruation is very risky. For girls: If you have sex with a boy or man who has STI you are likely to get a more serious infection. For boys: If the girl or woman is infected with HIV her menstrual blood will be rich with HIV viruses and you are likely to be infected.

Developmental changes for boys

Boys at this stage grow hair on their pubis, in their armpits and on their faces. They grow taller, their sex organs grow bigger, their voices change and become deeper, they become more muscular and their testicles start producing sperm. Boys start experiencing wet dreams and erections at puberty.

A young man in a sexual health workshop told the story below. If the story sounds familiar, it is because you are not alone. Many young people experience this because of lack of information about their developmental stages.

The story of George

I had my first wet dream when my parents and I were visiting my aunt. When I woke up in the morning realised that my underwear was wet and sticky. I quickly jumped out of bed and saw a wet mark on the sheet. I did not understand what was happening, but I felt so embarrassed about it. I quickly made the bed and changed into clean underwear. I took my wet underwear and put it in a plastic and pushed it between the wall and wardrobe. Fortunately it was our last day at her house, but my parents were so relaxed and not in a hurry to go home. This made me very anxious and restless, because I was afraid that my aunt would discover what I did to her sheet. I was so relieved when we finally left her house. I think she discovered what happened and informed my parents. My father called me and asked me about it, I was so embarrassed and scared that he might think badly of me. He told me that I probably had a wet dream and explained what it is all about. I think had I known about it before it happened it would have saved me all the embarrassment I experienced.

Boys who have reached puberty sometimes experience wet dreams. Wet dreams occur when a boy releases semen or ejaculates when he is asleep. You might notice this when you wake up in the morning find a wet sticky spot on your underwear or pyjamas. Wet dreams begin during puberty when the body starts making more testosterone (the hormone responsible for the formation of sperm). Almost all boys normally experience wet dreams at some stage during puberty and even as adults. Sometimes wet dreams can be embarrassing and confusing to young people, but it is completely normal. Try not to feel guilty about having wet dreams, because feeling guilty might lower your self-concept. Wet dreams are part of growing up and you cannot stop them from happening. It is also important to realise that wet dreams do not mean that you should have sex. They are part of your development.

Erections

Although erections in males happen from childhood, they sometimes cause a problem for young people when they happen in awkward places, for example, if you suddenly have an erection when you are at the stadium watching soccer.

An erection is the hardening of the penis that occurs when there is an increased blood flow to the penis causing it to enlarge and stand away from the body. It is difficult to urinate when you have an erection. Wait for it to go down before you try to urinate. Erections can be caused by sexual arousal or can happen for no reason. Erection occurs in males at all ages including babies and old men. Some people experience many erections in a day while some do not. It is normal, as people are different.

Sometimes teenagers worry that they are having too many erections or are embarrassed when an erection happens in an odd place. There is no reason to be embarrassed or to worry that something is wrong with you. Your body is acting naturally for a person of your age. Erections can also happen while you are asleep. The penis can become erect and go down about 5 to 7 times while you are asleep. It is normal.

> **Remember 2.6:** Wet dreams and erections are natural and normal. However, having wet dreams and erections is not a sign that you need to have sex. Wet dreams only happen when you are asleep and you cannot control them. You do not have to feel embarrassed about them. They are natural and part of your normal development.

To conclude this chapter, take a few minutes and read the poem below entitled "I love you my body".

I love you my body

You are like a plant that needs love, nurturing and care to grow to a beautiful tree.
You housed and protected my soul long before I was born.
You are the vehicle that brought me to this world.
Without you I wouldn't be here.
You are still and will still be doing all these things with love.
I love you my body!
Yes, till death do us part.

I am so happy that I have you as my body.
I wouldn't have chosen a better one.
Your love and warmth surrounds and protect me every day.

I cannot get tired of looking at your unique beauty.

When I stand in front of the mirror you always look at me and smile.

Your eyes give me a spark of encouragement to get out there and move on.

I move closer and kiss you and tell you how much I love you.

You simply smile at me.

Yes, it gives me pleasure to know that you are mine, mine alone.

I am the only one who has the right to touch you.

No one, I mean no one has the right to touch you without my
permission.

Yes, no one shall touch you because I know how and when to say "NO!"

I love you my beautiful body!

Yes, I know that I have a responsibility to look after you.

My parents/guardians have done their part it is now my turn.

I shall always love, nurture and care for you.

I shall try my best to protect you from trauma and disease.

If trauma and disease happen to get us, I will ensure that we get the
best treatment.

I shall never allow anyone to abuse you or me.

I shall never misuse you or allow anyone to misuse you.

I love you, my body. You are beautiful and unique.

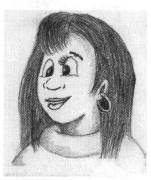

CHAPTER 3

WHAT ARE RELATIONSHIPS?

Introduction

Relationships are when people connect with others over a period of time. Relationships have the following characteristics: attachment, commitment and interdependence. Relationships are important in our lives because they give us a sense of belonging, security, identity, support, and meaning to our lives and happiness. People relate to each other in terms of their feelings, thoughts, physical reactions and actions.

Young people like other human beings, are social beings. They belong to a family, community, country and the world. They develop relationships with themselves, people around them, and the environment where they find themselves. There is a sense of interdependence among people who are in a particular relationship. In other words, people relate to each in order to achieve common goals or support the achievement of a set goal. In Xitsonga they say "munhu i munhu hi vanwana" (direct translation: a person is a person because of other people). This simply means that relationships are very important in people's lives. As human beings we are interdependent and need to relate to each other for survival. Very good- more of this will also be useful.

How you relate to other people and the environment around you depends on your feelings about yourself i.e. your relationship with yourself. If you love yourself and are happy about yourself you tend to have better relationships with other people. If you hate yourself or are unhappy with yourself, your relationship with other people will not be good.

You might sometimes have seen people kicking and cursing a stone because they are unhappy about something in their minds. This type of behaviour reflects what is happening inside that individual. It results from the conversation that the individual has with her/himself. Human beings spend a lot of time relating to themselves. This even happens when you are talking to other people. The relationship you have with yourself plays itself out when you relate to other people. For example, violent and abusive people are people who have a bad relationship with themselves. You need to build a good relationship with yourself in order to build good relationships with other people. If we can all develop a good relationship with ourselves, this world would be a better place to live in, free of violence and full of love.

There are different grades of relationships, distant and close. They also happen at different levels and in different contexts. Take a normal day in your life and think about the following questions. How many people do you relate to from the time you wake up in the morning to the time that you go to bed? What contribution do they make to your life? When we are at home we have relationship with our parents as a child, with brothers or sisters your siblings or grandson or granddaughter to your grandmother, etc. When you are at school you are a student to your teachers, a friend to your friends, a colleague to your fellow students, a boyfriend or girlfriend to your partner and so on. You get into a taxi you relate to fellow passengers. What is important in relationships is the association with each other. What happens if you do not relate to other people? You often get isolated, lonely and unhappy.

What skills do I need in order to have good relationships?

In order to have a good relationship you must first have a good relationship with yourself:

- Love and respect yourself.
- Always remember that you are on this earth for a purpose and you have a responsibility to fulfil that purpose, or your role on earth is meaningless.
- Feel good about yourself and always think positively.
- You need to be considerate and caring towards others. Make people around you feel that they are important.
- You need to be tolerant, respectful to and interested in other people.
- You need to be sincere, honest and open to yourself and other people you relate to i.e. your family, friends, partner and community. However, always allow yourself to continue being an individual.
- Make time for yourself and your own activities. This gives you an opportunity to relate to yourself.
- Ensure that you mix with people who affirm and love you.
- Always ask yourself what you want in a relationship and do not accept what you do not want. If you experience physical or emotional problems in your relationship with family, friends or partner, visit a counsellor or a health care provider to discuss your problems.

How do I maintain a good relationship with my family?

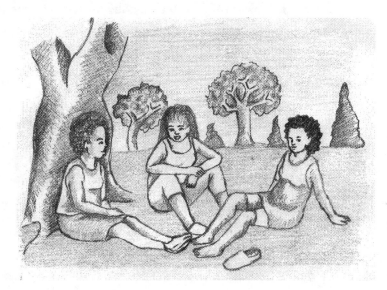

As a human being you are a unique individual who belongs to a unique family and has a relationship with self, family and society at large. We have discussed the importance of having a good relationship with yourself and now we will discuss the importance of having a good relationship with your family. If you want a good relationship with your parents, you need to:

- trust them, as you trust yourself;
- develop a caring attitude for the welfare and happiness of your family;
- show interest in your family members and be a good listener when they talk to you about themselves;
- be sincere and open to your family and let them know what you are.

If you want your family to trust you, you have to be truthful. When you talk to your parents be clear and specific about what you are saying. Also ensure that your family is aware of your feelings about what is happening within the family. Express your appreciation and affection to your family members. Develop and maintain a positive relationship with your sisters and brothers. Encourage mutual support during family crises. Show your parents that you are responsible by keeping your promises and facing the consequences of your actions. Know your rights and ensure that they are not violated. Another important thing in your relationship with your parents is to ask for forgiveness if you have wronged them and to forgive them if they make mistakes.

How do I maintain a good relationship with my friends?

Friendships are very important in people's lives especially young people. It is important to realise that friendships can occur across the sex, age, culture, language and race divides. You have probably heard your parents saying to you that you must choose your friends properly. It is important to choose friends because friends have a great influence on you, especially during your teenage years. The influence that friends have on you is referred to as peer pressure. Peer pressure is the pressure, stress or strain you feel from friends to act, behave, think and look in a particular way. Peer pressure can be good or bad for you. Good peer pressure is when you are encouraged to participate in good or healthy activities. It happens when your friends push you into something good that you did not have the courage to do, or were not even aware that you could do it. For example, your friends who have seen you play a particular sport and have realised that you are good at it, push you to join the team.

Bad peer pressure is when your friends coerce you into doing something that you did not want to do, because you know it is wrong. Bad peer pressure usually gets you into trouble with your family, school and the law. It is often difficult to resist peer pressure, but it can be done. What you can do is to try and pay more attention to your own feelings and use your inner strength and self-confidence to stand firm on your word. Resist doing what your friends want you to do when you know it is wrong.

To build a good friendship with your friends, try and make friends with people who have values that are similar to your own. Always try and be part of a group that allows you to be individuals with a right to think and make decisions for yourselves. As friends you need to be considerate and caring towards each other, i.e. to give and take on both sides. You need to be loyal, truthful and genuinely interested in each other. However, you need to be able to correct or guide each other when you realise that one of you is doing wrong things or misbehaving. You need to talk about your problems and share secrets. If your friend is poor and cannot afford a lunch box or "carry", share your lunch box with him or her.

You might have experienced another type of relationship where you find yourself having feelings that are much stronger than the feelings you have for your friends. Some people become restless or even tremble when they see this person or when they are in the company of this person. They also feel warmth, affection and the desire to kiss or touch him or her. If you have not yet experienced this, it is fine. You will get those feelings one day. The feelings that are talked about are feelings that happen when you are with your boyfriend or girlfriend or partner (as some people prefer to call it). These feelings are the beginning of a love relationship.

How do I know that I am really in love?

There is no simple answer to this question. Unfortunately with love you are the only one who can tell. What is discussed here is just to help you through. Firstly, make sure that you understand what love is. Many people view love as a relationship that is more intense than that which you feel for your friends. It is about believing that your partner is very important to you. Love is about caring, warmth, affection and desire for him or her.

Secondly, before you commit yourself to a relationship, you need to check your feelings again about this person. She/he must be a person you trust and feel comfortable with. You need to decide about how far you are prepared to go in this relationship, i.e. do you want to be intimate with her/him? Do not allow anyone to force you into a relationship if you are not ready or if you have doubts about the individual. Once you have made your decision about the relationship, be comfortable with it. Love means allowing each other to grow as individuals, commitment and loyalty. If you are not sure, it is a good idea to take your time before you commit yourself.

> **Remember 3.1:** Your ability to love and be loved depends on your sense of self-worth and self-esteem. You cannot truly love someone if you do not love, respect and accept yourself. Before you can love someone you need to learn to love yourself.

How do I maintain a good relationship with my partner?

As in all relationships, your ability to love your partner depends on your ability to love yourself. Your expression of love depends on your self-concept. You can only truly love your partner if you love, respect and accept yourself. Your relationship with your partner must be based on love. You need to learn to love yourself before you can experience true love.

In your relationship with your partner, there must be mutual respect (you value who the person is and you understand and never challenge her/his boundaries), trust, good communication, honesty, fairness and equality, support for each other in good and difficult situations and separate identities. Both of you support and respect each other's ideas, beliefs and wishes, no matter how different they are from your own. Neither of you use put-downs, guilt, shame, aggression, threats and silence, as tactics to get what you want and violate each other's rights. You value each other as friends and as individuals. You negotiate with each other on areas of disagreement.

> **Remember 3.2:** A positive relationship allows you to continue being your own person.
> A bad relationship is one in which you do not feel you can be yourself

What causes conflict between partners?

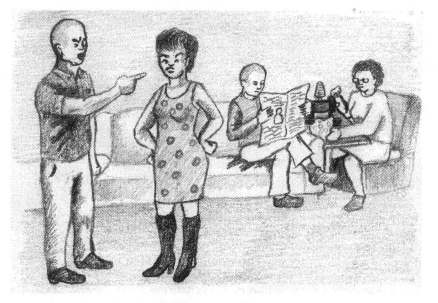

Disagreement between partners with no violence.

Conflicts arise in a relationship when the partners try to control and force each other to accept their point of view or do things their way. They can also arise when one partner gives too much and is always the one making sacrifices. As partners it is important to maintain a balance between giving and receiving.

When you find yourself in a conflict situation with your partner, try and identify the problem from both partners' perspective. Ensure that you are both clear about how you feel about the problem and to express this. You and your partner should listen carefully to each other's feelings and views. If your emotions are very strong, take a break to cool down. Find safe ways of getting rid of your anger and frustration. Work together and find out whether the problem is one of different values, beliefs and attitudes, or a practical issue. Avoid bringing complaints from the past because they can confuse issues. Do not try and force your partner to accept your solution if she/he is not satisfied. Do not humiliate your partner or use the incident as a power struggle.

Remember 3.3: If you are a man, you do not have to prove your manhood by making all decisions. You must never hit a girl or woman to show your manhood. Real men do not abuse or beat up girls and women. They give them love and care at all times.

CHAPTER 4

HOW DO I KEEP MYSELF HEALTHY?

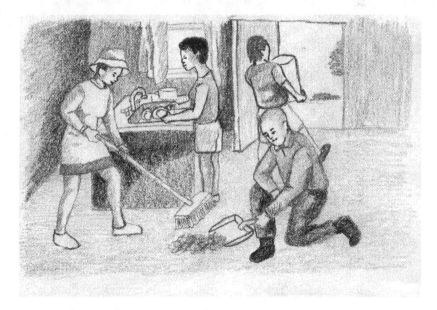

What does being healthy mean?

Health means different things to different people. Being healthy means different things to different people. What does being healthy mean to you? How do you consider yourself healthy or not healthy, and why? If you consider yourself healthy, what do you need to do to remain healthy? If you consider yourself unhealthy, what do you need to do to be healthy?

The concept "health" has been defined as a state of complete wellbeing that is physical, mental, social and spiritual. It does not only mean the absence of diseases or infirmity. To be healthy in this context means you have no physical, mental, emotional or social problems. As indicated in chapter 3, there are millions of germs that are attacking us every second and we also live with a lot of bacteria in our bodies. It is equally impossible to have a life that does not have emotional and social problems. What this definition is saying is that at all times we must try to move towards having a life that has no physical, emotional or social problems.

To be healthy you need to build a good relationship with yourself, your family, your teachers, colleagues, your friends and elders in your community. Being healthy means that you have self-esteem, and good relationships with yourself, family, partner and community. To have self-esteem you need to love yourself and believe in yourself. Take control of your life. It also means that you are able to deal with the changes in your body and your mind. You need time to relax and rest. Sleep for at least six hours per night.

As you have noticed, puberty causes all kinds of changes in your body. Your skin becomes oily very easily. At times you sweat for no reason and you might have noticed that there are odours where you never had them before, for example, armpits, feet and genitals. To cope with this wash your body with soap and water at least once a day. This will help wash away any bacteria that are contributing to the smell. Wash your hair every day if you kept it natural. Wash plaited hair and dreadlocks at least once a week or as advised by your hairdresser. Wear clean clothes, socks and underwear each day. It is a good idea to avoid sharing towels with other family members or friends, as infections can pass from person to person.

If you are concerned about the way your armpits smell, you can use a deodorant or an antiperspirant. If you choose to use a deodorant or antiperspirant, be sure to read the directions. If you are sensitive to this or develop an irritation, stop using it. If you cannot afford an antiperspirant, use bicarbonate of soda on your armpits. If you cannot afford that, use the traditional method: rub dry ashes into your armpits and wipe it off with a dry cloth before putting on your clothes. It is important to realise that if you wash every morning with soap and water it might not be necessary to use deodorants. Wash plaited hair and dreadlocks at least once a week or as advised by your hairdresser.

Try to avoid developing cracks in your skin or mucus membrane, to prevent the germs from gaining entrance into your body through those cracks. If you happen to have cracks use skin creams to treat them. If you have injuries to the skin, visit your nearest clinic for treatment.

Brush your teeth at least twice a day, in the morning and before you go to bed. Rinse your mouth after eating if possible. Visit the dentist or dental clinic at least once a year. If you have problems with your teeth, visit a dental clinic or dentist as soon as possible.

After using the toilet, clean yourself from the front of your private parts to the back. If you wipe to the front, you risk pulling germs from the anus to the vagina or urethra. Wash your hands after using the toilet, after blowing your nose, coughing, after touching animals and after gardening. It is also important to wash your hands after visiting a sick person at home or in hospital.

If you are a girl, you should never try to wash the inside of your vagina unless instructed by a health provider. Do not put anything in your vagina to try and dry it. Avoid using antiseptics and strong soaps on your private parts. During menstruation wash yourself at least twice a day to keep clean. Do not use deodorant or perfumes on your genitals. They can cause irritation Have regular Pap smears done, especially if you are sexually active. Do self-breast examinations every month after your menstrual period.

If you are a boy, wash your scrotum, behind the scrotum, between the scrotum and thighs and between buttocks every day. Also wash and clean the penis whether you are circumcised or not. If you are not circumcised, push back the foreskin and gently clean the glans area. Do monthly testicular self-examinations. (See chapter 6) and have your prostate gland checked by a doctor once a year, especially when you grow older.

1. Ensure that the water you drink is clean and safe for consumption. If you are not sure, boil it or add jik to the water to purify it. Add one teaspoon of Jik to 25 litres of water in container. Cover the container and let the water stand for at least two hours before use.
2. If you are on treatment, take your medication as prescribed.
3. Try to avoid accidents and injuries.
4. If you have any allergies, avoid areas or food or whatever causes the allergy.
5. Use condoms to provide protection against diseases and unwanted pregnancy.
6. Look after your body by maintaining good personal hygiene.
7. Look after your mind.
8. Always respect the right of control over your body.
9. Always maintain an equal balance of control and power in a sexual relationship.
10. Have access to information.

11. If you experience physical or emotional problems, visit your nearest clinic or discuss your problems with a health provider.

What can I do to maintain good hygiene in my environment?

We all have the responsibility of keeping our environment clean. An environment that is not clean attracts flies, which bring different diseases to our communities. Having a clean environment starts with you as an individual. Keep your environment clean and avoid littering. If you realise that your environment is dirty you can organise cleaning campaigns with your community.

What type of food must I eat in order to be healthy?

As a young person who is growing fast, you need a balanced diet. A balanced diet must consist of the following: carbohydrates, protein, vitamins, fats, fibre and water. As you might have noticed, it is sometimes very difficult to get all types of foods in each meal. It is even more difficult to have protein. However, it is still healthy to eat food that contains protein at least twice a week.

Carbohydrates or starch, are foodstuffs like pap, samp, bread, rice, potatoes, sweet potatoes, cassava, macaroni, spaghetti, noodles, sugar and bananas. Avoid eating more than one type of starch in any one meal, e.g. eating pap with potato chips. Carbohydrates give you energy. If the body takes in too much carbohydrates, it stores it as fat.

Proteins are foodstuffs like beef, eggs, fish, chicken, beans, bambaranuts, cowpeas, peanuts, pegeon-peas, milk, timongo/marula nuts, and peanut butter. Protein is necessary for the repair of worn-out tissues. Too much protein in your body is stored as fat. Lack of protein in your body can result in a disease called pellagra and children can suffer from kwashiorkor.

Vitamins need to be consumed daily, e.g. muroho/morogo, cabbage, carrots, beetroot, spinach, lettuce, cucumber, tomatoes, pumpkins, oranges, paw-paws, pineapples, apples, mangoes, bananas, pears and avocados.

Fibre, e.g. sorghum pap, tihove/samp, brown bread, apples, pears, whole wheat bread, is important for bowel movement and prevention of constipation.

Water is very important. You need to drink at least one litre of water every day. It prevents constipation and is essential for every bodily function. Water makes up between 60 and 80% of your body. Water cleans your body and keeps your skin healthy. Water also cleans your kidneys.

Fats. The body needs a little fat in order to absorb some vitamins. Too much fat results in weight gain. We get fat from meat, eggs and cheese.

Remember 4.1: Health is a right and as a right it should be available and affordable when you need it. You should be able to access it at all times. As a right always comes with responsibility, you are responsible for keeping yourself healthy at all times and to seek health assistance when the need arises. You have a responsibility to get and use information about health.

Exercise regularly

Exercise is very important for the functioning of your body. It is good for your heart, for the digestion of food and prevention of constipation. It also relieves stress and prevents heart problems. Exercise can be anything that makes muscles work hard and increases your breathing and heart rate, e.g. playing soccer, netball, basket ball, games that make you run around and jump, traditional dancing, walking for at least one kilometre per day, or pushing a wheelbarrow that is carrying a load that weighs at least 20kg. You are also exercising when you are carrying a heavy load on your head.

Exercise keeps our muscles supple and strong. It prevents heart diseases, weight problems and stress. Exercise increases the heart's ability to pump blood around the body to all muscles. Exercise makes the heart and lungs work harder and they start providing oxygen faster. Exercise strengthens our muscles, making it easier for them to repeat movements.

Avoid harmful practices

There are many young people who engage in practices that are harmful to themselves and others, e.g. boozing, driving under the influence of alcohol, taking or injecting drugs, prostitution, having sex without a condom, participating in crime and gangsterism. Engaging in these practices is very detrimental to your health and can expose you to unnecessary physical and emotional trauma and criminal activities.

Remember 4.2: There is nothing that can hinder you from leaving healthy
Believe in yourself. Love yourself and have a positive sense of belonging. Have a positive attitude towards yourself and others. Have a positive self image and self concept. Have a healthy mind and work hard to achieve your goals. Eat healthy and exercise regularly.

CHAPTER 5

I AM A VIRGIN

A virgin is a male or female who has never had penetrative sex or sexual intercourse. You can have a relationship but choose not to have penetrative sex with your partner. In this era of HIV and AIDS, many young people avoid penetrative sex until they are sure that they are both HIV negative.

Exercise 5: The story of John and Martin

Hey! Guys I have this big story for you come closer. Hey! I had it nice last night with this girl, hey! You know her, man. Hey! John and Marvin get out of here I am not talking to you man. I do not share these big stories with virgins you know. Get out of my sight, super virgins!

If you were John or Marvin, how would you have reacted to this kind of treatment?
What skills would you use to deal with the situation?

The story above is a good example of negative peer pressure. John and Martin's friend is using bullying tactics to pressure them into having sex when they know that they are not ready. When faced with such a situation you use your assertive skills, good self-concept and inner strength to help you to walk away from this type of situation.

Many young people who choose to be virgins come under a lot of pressure from friends who do not approve of their decision. They humiliate them and make them feel inadequate. It is this pressure that can get you into trouble because you want to please your friends. Nobody wants to feel left out of things. Some people might feel that they have to lose their virginity to keep up with their friends or to be accepted. Although many young couples do not pressure each other to submit to sex, it happens that in a relationship one person wants to have sex and the other does not. A situation like this can be a source of stress and strain on their relationship. If faced with such situations, you need to do what is right for you and not anyone else. It is sometimes difficult for young people to negotiate in such situations because they do not know what to say because of lack of assertive skills.

You need to stand up for your rights and respect the rights of others. Express what you believe, feel and want in a direct and honest way. You need to have skills to deal with such pressures. You need to have the assertive and communication skills, which are discussed in chapter 1.

The decision to have sex or not to have sex is a choice that is different for everyone. If you have made your choice to be sexually active, respect your friends' choice. There are many young people who choose to remain virgins until they find the right person. Do not allow yourself to be pressured into having sex when you are not ready.

It is important to think seriously about what you believe and feel about sex as well as considering the impact that becoming sexually active will have on your relationship with your partner. Never allow yourself to be pushed into doing something that does not feel right for you. You should only have a sexual relationship if this is what you want, not because everyone is doing it or because your partner or friends are putting pressure on you.

Some young people postpone their first sex, because they are thinking more carefully about what it means to lose their virginity and begin a sexual relationship. Some wait longer before having their first sex, because:

- they don't want an unplanned pregnancy;
- they are protecting themselves from STI and HIV and AIDS;
- of their religious beliefs;
- They realise that they are not emotionally ready for sex.

It is fine if you decide to put off sex, no matter what anyone says. Being a virgin is one of the things that prove you are in charge, and that you are powerful enough to make your own decisions about your body.

> **Remember 5.1:** It is only you, who can decide when the time is right for you to become sexually active. Having sex to impress your friends will not make you feel good about yourself in the long run. True friends do not care whether you are a virgin or not. They respect your decision.

How can I enjoy sex without penetration or sexual intercourse?

Exercise 6: A letter written to the editor of a magazine

Dear editor

My partner and I have been together for about a year now. We are still virgins and love each other so much and spend most of our time together. We kiss, talk, laugh, hold hands, study and play games together sometimes until late in the evening and thereafter he just walks me home. We both feel that we are not yet ready for sex. How are we going to know when we are ready?

Firstly, decide whether it is right for you to become sexually active. Making this decision is one of the most important decisions you will ever make in your life. Secondly, make up your own mind about whether your partner is the person you want to have your first sex experience with and when it will be the right time for you to be sexually active. You also need to find out from your partner whether he/she is ready for sex. Finally, it is important to realise that sex has very serious emotional consequences. You need to consider your feelings and the consequences of sex before you engage in sexual intercourse e.g. your personal and religious beliefs, the possibility of pregnancy and STIs.

There are many ways of getting sexual satisfaction without penetration. These are used by both virgins and sexually active people. Virgins use these methods to delay their first sexual penetrative sex. While sexually active people use them as variation in their sexual activities. These methods are also good for the prevention of HIV and AIDS.

- Masturbation and mutual masturbation **(discussed below);**
- Kissing, caressing and sharing the body;
- Massage;
- Hugging and cuddling;
- Thigh sex (rubbing the penis on the woman's thighs with no ejaculation taking place on the inner side of her thighs);
- Body sex (rubbing the penis on the woman's body);
- Pillow sex or sex talk (Sharing your sexual fantasies);
- Reading erotic books or watching sexy movies together.

Before you engage in any of the above-mentioned sexual activity, make sure that you are ready and that your partner is ready for it. If your partner is not comfortable or not ready, do not force or coerce her/him into doing something she/he does not want. You can also stop these sexual activities if you want to, or if you are uncomfortable with it. If you partner says "NO" during non-penetrative sex, stop immediately. You also have the right to say "NO" if you do not want to continue with the sexual activity.

Masturbation

Masturbation is a mixture of sexual feeling and intimacy. It involves stimulating yourself or your partner stimulating you to excitement and satisfaction. Many people, both boys and girls, experience their first orgasm through masturbation. It helps people to discover what really turns them on. There is no need to feel guilty when you masturbate. Many people feel guilty because as children they were told not to touch or explore themselves. Although some people often regard masturbation as not right, it is a normal process that everyone goes through. Masturbation in girls starts a little later than in boys.

Mutual masturbation is when you and your partner masturbate each other. It is when your partner is doing what you usually do to yourself. It can include kissing, caressing and massage.

Remember 5.2: It is ok to wait as long as you want before having sex. The decision is yours to make and it is going to be yours to live with, so make sure it's the right decision. You cannot die of sexual stimulation or an erection. You cannot go mad or become sterile if you do not have sex or you are refused sex. Do not be tricked into sex by a person who tells these stories.

CHAPTER 6

I AM SEXUALLY ACTIVE

Exercise 7: Joyce's story

Thembi: Hi! Joyce.

Joyce: Hey girls listen to this virgin she calls me by name. Hey! Virgin girl, I am not Joyce to you, ok! I am Rejoice's mother ok! You will call me Joyce when you know what a man is.

Pinkie: Joyce that is not a good way of talking to Thembi! She was just greeting you. Is it wrong to greet?

Joyce: Oh! Hey! Pinkie who invited you into this conversation? Anyway I do not know why you are also keeping that little thing of yours shut! God gave you that thing to use. You must go to the labour room and feel what other women are feeling.

Pinkie: You know what Joyce, you chose to be a mother and we have accepted it. But it seems as if it difficult for you to accept that we chose to remain virgins. Why are you always uncomfortable with our decision? We have never said bad things to you, because you are our friend.

Joyce: (Just shrugs her shoulders and leaves).

Joyce (Thinking): I really envy these girls. I feel so bad about my situation; I am the only one in this school who has a child. I hate being a mother! But, when I am with them I will make them believe that I enjoy being a mother. I will always talk about my daughter. Yaa! I also want them to feel what I feel inside.

Questions

1. What is Joyce's problem?
2. How would you describe her relationship with the other girls?
3. Does it happen in real life situations?
4. What do you think she wants to achieve by her actions?
5. What skills does she need to deal with her situation?

To be sexually active must be your choice and it is also your choice to stop being sexually active. It must also be your partner's choice to be sexually active and it also your partner's choice to stop having sex. You have a right to say "NO" to sex and your partner also has the same right. You cannot be forced into having sex and you cannot force your partner into having sex with you. Anyone who forces you or continues to have sex with you even when you have said "NO" to sex has violated your rights and can be charged with rape. If you force or ignore your partner when he/she says "NO" to sex, you have violated their rights and you will be charged with rape.

Take a few minutes and think about your situation and try to answer the following questions: Was it your choice to have a sexual relationship? What do you want to achieve by being sexually active? Do you still want to continue to be sexually active? If you do not want to, do you want to stop? Do you enjoy a sexual relationship with your partner?

If it is your choice to be sexually active, then you have a right to enjoy sex. For you to enjoy sex ensure that your partner is participating in it, because he or she chose to participate. You must not coerce your partner into sex, because you will not enjoy it. Make sure that your partner is comfortable with your choice. Communication is very important in relationship and sex, because good sex is about mutual sharing and enjoyment. You need to decide as a couple on the type of sexual relationship that you want to enjoy - penetrative or non-penetrative sex. You can enjoy sex without penetration **(see chapter 5).**

For sex to be satisfying for both partners, both need to take responsibility for their own fulfilment. You need to tell or show each other what you like and what you do not like; what you would like differently, and what you would like to try out. Good sex involves much more than just intercourse. It involves all the senses, smell, touch, taste, sound and sight as well as our own emotions. If you are tense, self-conscious or anxious, you cannot relax and enjoy the experience.

If your partner truly loves you, she or he will not push or pressure you to do something you do not believe in or aren't ready for yet. But at the same time, don't beat yourself up or be too hard on yourself if you have sex and then wish you hadn't. Having sexual feelings is normal and handling them can sometimes be difficult to do.

Just because you had sex once does not mean you have to continue or say 'yes' later. If you did not like it you can still stop having sex if it is your choice. Do not continue to be sexually active just because you tried it once. Making mistakes is human and it is a major part of development and you can learn from your mistakes.

NB: Read chapter 8 to learn more about sexual relationships that are wrong and punishable by law.

> **Remember 6.1:** Having sex to impress your friends will not make you feel good about yourself in the long run. True friends do not really care whether you are a virgin or not; they respect your decision and love you for who you are. Forcing someone to have sex with you when they have said "NO" is a crime.

Contraception

The decision to have or not to have a baby when you are in a relationship is very crucial. If you do not want to have a baby, you need to use contraceptives. Some people prefer using double methods, e.g. a condom and a contraceptive. This makes both partners take responsibility. The decision we make about whether or when we want to have children depends on who we are and who we wish to become. If you are still at school and have aspirations of becoming a professional one-day, you might choose to postpone having children because it might interfere with your education. In that case you might consider using contraceptives or abstaining from sex until you are both ready.

Methods of contraception

There are several methods that you can choose from, hormonal, spermicides, barrier methods and emergency contraceptive pill.

Hormonal methods change the way your body functions. They suppress the development of eggs or change the cervical mucus so that it can be hostile to the sperm or affecting the walls of the womb and make it impossible for the fertilised egg to implant. Hormonal methods include injectables, pill and implants. Emergency contraceptive pills commonly known as morning after pills are contraceptives that can be used to prevent pregnancy following an unprotected sexual intercourse. They contain some hormones and are used within 72 hours of unprotected sexual intercourse. Emergency contraceptive pill will not protect you from HIV, AIDS and STIs.

The barrier methods include diaphragms, cervical caps and condoms. The diaphragm and cervical cap are not available in the public institutions. The male condom is readily available, but the female condom is hard to get. There are also spermicides that kill the sperm before it can fertilise the egg.

Another method that can be used is the intra-uterine contraceptive device (IUCD). There two types, the loop and the copper T. The loop prevents the egg from implanting because it fills the uterus. The copper T emits copper that kills the sperm. There is also sterilisation for men and women. These are permanent methods where the female fallopian tubes are tied and cut to prevent the sperm from meeting the egg. In males it is called a vasectomy, and the tubes coming from the testicles are tied and cut to prevent the sperm from moving to the urethra.

Remember 6.2: You can prevent getting pregnant by using contraceptives. Using a condom will protect you from HIV and AIDS.

Exercise 8: I am pregnant or my girl friend is pregnant

"Oh! God, hear my prayer. I don't know what to do. I cannot tell my mother or my sister they will die if they can hear my story. I talk to Jim about it and he

decided to disappear. He does not even talk to me when we meet in the library. Oh! God you know what he said, "Don't mess-up with my life. Don't go around telling people you are carrying my baby. You know it's not me who impregnated you; you must be having other guys on campus. Anyway why didn't you use contraceptives? Yesses, you freshers are trouble, you know!" Yes, it would be a scandal for a first year student to claim sexual relationships with the SRC vice president. Sometimes I want to die and disappear from the face of this earth. Oh! God I seem to be gaining weight everyday! This thing is growing in me. No it is not a thing it is my child, I can feel it moving. What must I do! I am stuck! I know when I get home my parents are going to be mad at me. Yes, I wasted their money. They brought me to this prestigious university to study law not to make babies. I have disappointed them. Oh! God what must I do. I hate myself; yes it is my fault. I should not have listened to him when he said condoms are not good for virgins they give them AIDS. He lied to me and I was a fool to listen to him. Oh! God what must I do!"

- What is the problem?
- What skills does she need in order to deal with this problem?
- What does being pregnant mean to you?
- Is your pregnancy planned or unplanned?
- Given this situation, what steps would you take to deal with the problem?
- How would you support a friend or girlfriend who wants to terminate her pregnancy?

To be pregnant means you are now going to be a mother; or if your girlfriend is pregnant it means you are going to be a father. It means that you are now expected to provide for the needs of your baby. There are many young people in our country that become fathers and mothers when they are not yet ready for it.

There are many reasons that contribute to this: lack of knowledge about how their bodies work; lack of sexuality education; peer pressure; myths; rape; and sexual abuse by relatives. In some cases, parents pressurise their daughters to have children in order to get the child support grant. And this is wrong. In many communities young people are told not to have sex and not to fall pregnant or make a girl pregnant, without giving them the information and skills on how to prevent it. Giving them information about sexuality would empower them to make informed choices.

Many young people indulge in sexual activities just because everyone in their school or community is sexually active. The results of such sexual activity, which might be pregnancy or diseases, come as a shock to many of them. They are often blamed and labelled as promiscuous. It is worse for girls, because some are rejected by their families and sometimes dumped at their partner's home. More often than not, their partners also reject them, calling them names and even denying having sex with them. It is experiences like this that lowers the self-confidence and self-esteem of many young people, making them hate themselves.

It is very unfortunate that there are no support services for young women who find themselves in this kind of crisis. There are no counsellors for young pregnant women and no support from either home or school, or educational institution. According to the South African policy, pregnant girls have the right to continue with their education when they are pregnant. However, many of them drop out because of harassment from their peers in the classroom, or from the school itself and teachers. During crisis times like this you need support from your friends and adults around you. If you find yourself in a similar position, or know a friend who is, it is important to go for emotional support and counselling. Try and accept your peers who are going through this problem. Do not be judgmental and reject them.

If your pregnancy is planned, you need to visit a health provider for antenatal care. You are expected to attend antenatal clinics until you have your baby. The antenatal clinics prepare parents-to-be for labour and for care of the baby. You need to decide as a couple where you are going to deliver your baby, and whether you want to be together during delivery. Prepare yourselves socially and psychologically for the baby. You need to realise that you will have to make serious adjustments to your lives to accommodate the newcomer. If you are working, you also need to make arrangements for the care of your child when you are both at work.

If your pregnancy is unplanned, you need to decide whether to continue with the pregnancy or not. You need to decide whether you tell your partner and parents about it or not. If you have told your partner, what was his reaction? Know your rights. If you want to go through with the pregnancy, what does it mean to you and your future? How are you going to provide for your baby? If you plan not to go through with it, visit your clinic for information about the termination of pregnancy. The health workers have an obligation to give you information on where to get assistance. At the clinic or hospital where termination of pregnancy is performed, they will first have a counselling session with you before it is performed, and another one after the termination. Termination of pregnancy is very private and you do not need parental or your partner's approval for it. Remember that it is your body and you are the only one who has any right over it.

Remember 6.3: There are many ways of preventing unwanted pregnancy. Do not fall pregnant just because your friends have children or your friends are getting the child support grant. Having a child is a life-long commitment. Are you ready for it? Think of your future before you decide on being pregnant.

CHAPTER 7

WHAT INFECTIONS OR DISEASES CAN I GET IF I AM SEXUALLY ACTIVE?

Exercise 9: I am not feeling very well
Tick -tick, tick -tick

Lorraine: Hello, Maggie.

Maggie: Lorraine you sound awful, what is wrong?

Lorraine: I am not feeling well you know since James's departure on Tuesday.

Maggie: Hmm! You miss him aren't you?

Lorraine: Yes I do! But what I feel is not related to that. I think I felt it before he left, but I thought I was catching flu. But it seems, as if it is getting serious you know. I have this smelly discharge and lower abdominal pains. When I wee-wee it is so painful you know. I am scared Maggie, I think I am having an STI. I think my James is cheating on me.

Maggie: Lorraine, I am on my way I am taking you to the doctor right away. Is it ok?

There are many infections that come with sexual activity and these infections are collectively known as sexually transmitted infections (STIs), e.g. gonorrhoea, syphilis, candidiasis, Chlamydia, cancer, HIV and AIDS. These diseases will not be discussed in details. Visit your clinic for more information on the diseases.

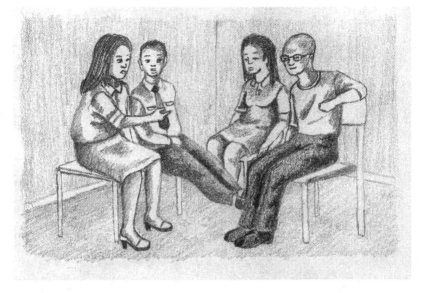

What are Sexually Transmitted Infections (STIs)?

STIs are diseases that are passed from one person to the other through sexual intercourse. If you find yourself having any of the signs and symptoms listed in the table below, visit a health provider. You could be having a sexually transmitted disease. STIs can be treated effectively if appropriate treatment is taken. Your partner also needs treatment. You need to abstain from sex during the treatment until all the symptoms have cleared.

Table: Signs of sexually transmitted infections

Females	Males
1. Unusual discharge from your vagina	Discharges from the end of the penis
2. Strong smelly discharge	Strong smelly discharge
3. Pain, burning or itching around the vagina	Pain during when urinating
4. Lower abdominal pain and pain in the back	Lower abdominal pain and pain in the back Fever or chills, headaches, general tiredness
5. Fever or chills, headaches, general tiredness	Sores or blisters on the genitals or mouth
6. Sores or blisters on the genitals or mouth	Genital warts
7. Genital arts	Swelling around the groin or swollen glands
8. Rashes or bumps on your body	Pubic lice or genital scabies
9. Pubic lice or genital scabies	

How can I protect myself from sexually transmitted infections?

- Say "No" to unprotected sex.
- Stick to one partner.
- Do not have sex with a stranger or someone you do not know very well.
- Use a condom when you have sex.
- Visit your clinic or doctor if you suspect that you have an STI.
- Tell your partner if you think you have an STI.
- Both you and your partner should have appropriate treatment.
- Do not have sex until you have finished your treatment and the symptoms have disappeared.

What is Human Immunodeficiency Virus **(HIV) and** Acquired Immunodeficiency Syndrome **(AIDS)?**

You are probably aware that South Africa has the largest number of people living with HIV and AIDS in the whole world, estimated at 4.2 million people with young people constituting the highest percentage. It is also estimated that 16 percent of young people between 15 and 19 and 1 in 4 women between the age of 20 and 29 years are HIV positive. The incidence of HIV and AIDS in South Africa is expected to increase drastically if measures are not taken to prevent the spread of HIV. It is clear that South Africa needs the contribution and effort of all South Africans, as individuals and communities, to prevent the spread of this disease. Let us all join hands and win the fight.

AIDS is an illness caused by a virus called the Human Immunodefiency Virus (HIV). HIV is a retrovirus, which attacks and destroys the body's immune system. For a person to get AIDS, the virus has to get into your blood. When a person first contracts the virus they show no symptoms of the disease, although they are carrying the virus and are HIV positive. Once someone shows signs it means that the virus has destroyed the body's ability to fight infections. More and more infections and illnesses will begin to occur.

How is HIV passed from one person to another?
The virus gets into the human body through unprotected sexual intercourse, contaminated needles and from mother to child during pregnancy and delivery. When you are HIV positive, you carry the virus in the blood, semen, vaginal secretion and breast milk. The virus can only be transmitted when you come into contact with the body fluids

of an infected person. You can get HIV by having sex with an infected person, sharing a needle with an infected person, being born of a mother who is infected or drinking breast milk from an infected woman. HIV cannot be transmitted through mosquito bites, coughing, sneezing, sharing eating utensils, sharing bathrooms, toilet seats, or hugging and kissing.

How do I know that I am living with HIV?

You might not be able to tell that you are infected until you have been tested. It is therefore important for all of us to have regular HIV testing in order to learn about our HIV status and protect ourselves and others. The testing process is referred to as voluntary counselling and testing (VCT). It is readily available in clinics and hospitals free of charge. Remember, you may be infected and totally healthy and may continue living for many years without showing any symptoms, but you are infectious. Some people have no symptoms until their immune system is damaged and opportunistic diseases start occurring. Some people get fever, headaches, sore muscles and joints, skin rashes, swollen lymph glands for one or two weeks. Some are usually discovered when they present with diseases such as TB, pneumonia, fungal infections and repeated STIs.

How can I protect myself against HIV and AIDS?

The first thing you need to know to protect yourself is that HIV and AIDS exists and there is no cure for it. Secondly you need to know how it is transmitted from person to person in order to take the proper measures to protect yourself. Lastly you can prevent yourself from getting HIV by:

- abstaining from sex;
- using a condom every time you have sexual intercourse (vaginal, anal or oral sex);

- Undergoing voluntary testing before you can indulge in sex. Choosing to have HIV test can be difficult decision. Discuss your decision with a counsellor before you take a test;

- Ensuring that your partner is also free of the virus by making sure she or he is tested, before having unprotected sex. However, it is possible for a person to be negative whilst they have the virus and can transmit it to their partners. This is called the window period;

- stick to one partner;

- always using a condom if you know that your partner is having other sexual partners;

- avoiding having sex with a person you do not know;

- avoiding casual sex;

- not injecting drugs;

- Using sex without penetration methods because there will not be any exchange of body fluids. (See in chapter 5)

I am HIV positive what do I need to do to live longer?

Accept your condition and allow your family to give you support by disclosing your condition. Remember you are not obliged to disclose. Many people living with HIV are discriminated against – be ready to experience such rejections.

- Maintain good personal hygiene.
- Stay in a well-ventilated room.
- Avoid over-crowded places.
- Eat a well balanced diet and use garlic and ginger in your diet.
- Avoid eating fermented foods and milk products.
- Take immune boosters or antiretroviral drugs as prescribed by your doctor.

- If you are on other treatment, take your medication as prescribed and complete your course
- Exercise.
- Avoid smoking and drinking.
- Get enough rest and relaxation.
- Get medical care if you are ill or if you see any signs of infection.
- Practice safer sex.
- Get emotional help if you realise you are not coping with your emotions as well as you would like to.
- Think positively. Remember that being HIV positive does not mean death. You can live with the virus for many years.
- Use a condom at all times to prevent getting STIs and reinfecting yourself.
- Avoid stress and learn to relax.

> **Remember 7.1:** HIV and AIDS is a reality. There is no treatment for it yet. However, to be HIV positive does not mean you have AIDS and death. It means you have the virus in your blood. If you look after yourself properly you can live with it for many years.

Cancers affecting the reproductive system

What is cancer?

The human body is made up of many living cells that form the different parts and systems of the body. Normally body cells grow, divide into new cells, and die in an orderly way. Sometimes the cells in a part of the body start growing out of control and become cancer. Unlike normal cells, cancer cells do not die they continue to grow and form new, abnormal cells that grow into other tissues, something that normal cells cannot do.

Cancer cells go on making new cells that the body does not need. These cells then spread to other parts of the body, where they begin to grow and form new tumors or growths that replace normal tissue. There are different types of cancers and they behave very differently in the human body. They also grow at different rates and respond to different types of treatments. Although cancer spreads to different part of the body, it is always gets its name from the place where it started.

There are many cancers that can affect male and female, but we are just going to discuss the cancers that affect the reproductive system. You are not likely to get these cancers as a young person. However, what you do now might put you at risk or save you from getting these cancers later in your life.

What cancers affect the reproductive system of a woman?

There are two common cancers that affect the female reproductive system. These are cancer of the breast and cancer of the cervix.

Cervical cancer

Cancer of the cervix is caused by the human papillomma virus, which is found in the semen of men. The virus attaches itself to the cervical cells. If the cervical cells are still growing it changes the shapes of the growing cells therefore resulting in abnormal cells that become cancerous.

Cervical cancer is commonly found in people who became sexually active very early in their lives, had children very early and also in those women who have had many children. Having multiple partners, weakened immune system, recurring STI, smoking, multiple pregnancies and poor nutrition can also contribute towards getting cancer.

Signs of cancer of the cervix are: lower abdominal pain, unusual vaginal bleeding, unusual vaginal discharge, and pain or bleeding after sex.

Cervical cancer can be treated if discovered at an early stage of its development. It can be discovered very early by doing a Pap smear. You can do Pap or cervical smears at a clinic or hospital, or at a private clinic or doctors consulting rooms.

What I do to reduce the risk of getting cervical cancer?

There are several simple steps that you can take to reduce the risk of developing cervical cancer:

- Get vaccinated against HPV. The HPV vaccine provides protection against the four types of HPV that are most commonly associated with cervical cancer and genital warts.
- Do pap smears regularly
- Practicing safe sex
- Stick to one partner
- Be a Non-Smoker

What is the human papillomavirus (HPV)?

The human papillomavirus (HPV) is the most common sexually transmitted infection. HPV is transmitted through:

- Sexual intercourse
- Genital-to-genital contact (i.e. No penile penetration is needed to contract the virus)
- Skin-to-skin contact with an infected person
- Touching the genitals of an infected partner and then your own
- Sharing sex toys without cleaning them properly first

How can I protect myself from getting infected with HPV?

Abstinence from all sexual activity is the only real method of prevention. There are also other ways that you can use to reduce the risk of getting infected with HPV:

- Get vaccinated against HPV. The HPV vaccine provides protection against the four types of HPV that are most commonly associated with cervical cancer and genital warts. It does not protect you against all known types of HPV.
- use condoms
- stick to one partner;
- Practicing safe sex
- Use gloves when touching someone's genitals
- Visit your doctor to find out if you are not infected and if you are not infected get vaccinated against HPV.
- Many countries including South Africa are routinely giving vaccinations against HPV to all girls at the age of nine years. Some countries are also vaccinating boys against this virus.

Breast cancer

Breast cancer is a group of cancer cells that start growing in the breast and spread to surrounding tissues and other parts of the body. Breast cancer is another cancer that is increasing in many countries including South Africa. It can also be treated if it is discovered in time. It is important for a young person to learn the techniques of examining her breast every month. This is called self-breast examination.

Breast Self Examination (BSE)

Stand in front of the mirror and inspect your breast for any abnormal signs. Check for any difference in the shape of your breasts and in the colour of the skin or nipples. Gently squeeze the nipples. Raise your hands and look at the breast from the side. Lie on your back. Using the pads of your fingers, feel each breast by making circular movements, starting from the outside and moving in towards the nipple. Make sure that you feel the whole breast. If you see or feel a lump or any dents or dimples in your breasts see a health care provider.

Signs of breast cancer

- Persistent pain in the breast or pain during menstruation.
- A lump in the breast. However not all lumps are cancers; many of them are harmless.
- Discharge from the nipples.
- Changes in the skin of the breast, such as dimpling.
- Changes in the nipples.
- Sores or swelling of the breast.
- Visit your health provider.

What cancers can affect the male reproductive organs?

There are two main cancers that affect the reproductive system of men, testicular cancer and prostate cancer. Since prostate cancer affects mature men, it will not be discussed in this book.

Testicular cancer

Testicular cancer or cancer of the testes, is a group of cancer cells that start growing in the in the testicles. It is more common among people between 15 and 35 years of age. Like any other cancer, testicular cancer is curable if discovered early. Young men need to perform a self-testicular examination every month.

Testicular self-examination

You can do the examination immediately after washing in warm water or any time when the testicles are relaxed. Inspect your scrotum, penis and groin for sores, discoloration, warts, cracks and swelling. If you notice any lumps, or swelling, or skin discoloration, or pain in the penis, scrotum or groin, visit your doctor or clinic. You might have realised that one testicle is slightly larger than the other is, it is normal. Place your thumbs over the testicle with the index and middle finger of each a hand behind the testicle. Examine one testicle at a time by gently rolling it between the fingers. The testicle should feel smooth and regular. Visit your health provider if you feel any lumps, pain or notice any changes in the size of the testicles.

Signs of testicular cancer

- Enlarged painless testicular lump.
- Occasionally there can be pain.
- Enlarged testicle.
- A feeling of heaviness or sudden accumulation of fluid in the scrotum.
- A dull ache in the lower abdomen or groin.
- Enlargement or tenderness of the breasts.

Remember 7.2: You can prevent yourself from getting STI and HIV and AIDS if you practice safe sex methods. If you happen to have STI, get treatment and ensure that your partner or partners are treated. Cancer can be prevented if you carry out self-examination and other early cancer detection tests.

CHAPTER 8

WHAT IS GENDER-BASED VIOLENCE?

You have probably heard or read about gender discrimination and gender based violence. In many countries discriminatory practices on the basis of being a female or male prevail in many situations where men and women find themselves. There many young people who have been subjected to gender discrimination and gender-based violence.

What is gender?

Exercise 10

In one workshop, participants were asked to think of the first day they realised that they were different from the opposite sex and how they felt about it. Here are some of their responses.

Facilitator: *Think of the first day you realise you were different from the opposite sex. How old were you? What was happening or what happened? How did you feel about it?*

Pule: *I was 8 years old when my father bought me my first bicycle. When he got home he called me and gave me the bike and said, "I will teach you how to ride it son". My sister who was 12 years old asks him where her bike was. My dad said, "Bikes are not for girls I brought you a beautiful doll". I felt so happy. I think my sister was not happy because she took her doll and went to her room and did not come out for dinner.*

Liana: *I was 6 years old on my first day at school. I wanted a toilet and so one and I just went in. It was a boy's toilet. As I was entering the door a boy just pushed me and said this is not a girl's toilet. Go to the girl's toilet on the other side. I felt so bad, because at the pre-school we used the same toilets. I did not understand why I should use a different one now.*

Doris: *I think I was 5 years old. I was with my father, carrying my younger brother on my back. We were rushing to the bus stop. My father was walking very fast and I asked him to take my younger brother because he was quite heavy for me. My father said firmly, where have you seen a man carrying a child? You are a girl it is your responsibility to carry him.*

Mpumi: *I realised that I was different from girls when we were urinating. Girls used to squat when urinating and boys used to stand. When we competed on how far our urine could go I used to win. I felt great about it.*

Hlanganani: *I learnt about it when my breasts started budding. My mother bought me a beautiful bra and told me to wear it and cover my breasts. She also showed me her beautiful bras. I was so happy.*

She told me that I am now growing up to being a beautiful young woman.

Ranisa: *I do not know how to say this, however I will tell you. I know that I was different from men when I was six years old. My uncle who was living with us raped me when my parents were not at home. I felt so bad and ashamed of myself.*

Joe: *I was 11 years old when we visited my grandmother who lives in the village. I was used to playing with my two sisters. When we were at my grandmother's home, she told me to stop playing with girls and go out with other boys to look after the goats and play games that will make me strong. I felt so bad.*

Try to answer the question asked by the facilitator.

What we gathered from the stories are two things, the biological difference between boys and girls and the discrimination that follows because of their biological difference. It is unequal treatment of someone based on their sex. Gender discrimination refers to any situation where a person is denied an opportunity or misjudged solely on the basis of their sex.

The discrimination between boys and girls (men and women) that is based on social roles that society has prescribed for them is referred to as gender. For example, a father who refuses to carry his own son, because he is a man – women however young they could be must be the ones carrying babies on their backs. Girls do not ride bicycles, they play with dolls. Boy told to go and do boys' work. Another important thing to note is that the feelings that were caused by the discrimination on the person discriminated upon were more intense than the feelings caused by realising the biological difference.

Take a few minutes and think about the following questions:

- What is the impact of this gender discrimination on the self-concept of the individual who is discriminated against? Discrimination lowers the self-concept of the person and therefore making that individual vulnerable to abuse.

- Let us take Pule's story, what impact do you think the incidence had on him? It gave him a feeling of greatness. He felt he is much better than his sister (a superiority complex) and that boosted his self-concept while the same incidence destroyed his sister's self-confidence and made her feel inferior. A superiority complex like inferiority complex is not good. It leads to hostile and oppressive attitudes towards people you perceive you are superior to them. An attitude of equality with other people makes you feel good about yourself and others.

- Try and put yourself in Ranisa's situation, how would you feel? You would definitely feel angry, ashamed and dirty. The story of Ranisa is common in South Africa.

- What do you think the incidents did to Ranisa's self-concept? It is true your self-concept would be destroyed.

- In your own view, what should be done to such people? Yes, they should be reported, arrested and stay in jail, because they will do the same thing to many other children.

As already indicated this unacceptable discrimination between women and men is referred to as gender discrimination. Gender are characteristics, roles and behaviour patterns that society has prescribed for men and women not because of their biological, but the cultural meanings that are given to the biological and physiological events that influence people's behaviour. Gender dictates how boys and girls must look, think, act and perceive the world they live in. Gender assigns characteristics like beauty for women and strength for men and these determines how boys and girls should be brought up. Good examples of this are in the story of Hlanganani and Joe.

What is gender-based violence?

Gender based violence is any act or behaviour that result in physical, sexual and emotional harm or suffering to girls and women. Gender violence includes among others physical abuse, emotional abuse, sexual abuse, sexual harassment, forced prostitution. Perpetrators of gender based violence can be family members, parents, friends, teachers, boyfriends, girlfriends and strangers.

1. Physical abuse

Physical abuse is includes the following: Burnt with a cigarettes or iron or stove or heater or candle or fire, beaten, pinched, made to work for no pay, stabbed, cut, suffocated, strangulated, drowned, made to sleep in the cold, not taken for treatment when sick. Physical abuse happens to both male and females.

2. Emotional abuse

Physical abuse refers to when a person is called names, insulted, sworn at, humiliated, threatened, bullied, denied food, my belongings taken away from me, treated differently from the others, always singled out for hard work and risky jobs, talking bad about you, talking bad about my people or people I love and when a person always brings up the mistake you made. Emotional abuse can happen to both men and women.

3. Sexually abused and sexual harassment

Sexual abuse and harassment can happen to both females and males. Sexual abuse includes: rape, touching your private parts without your consent, touching your bottom, touching or fondling your breasts, forced to kiss someone, forced to have sex with someone, forced to have sex with an animal, made to strip and parade naked in front of someone or a group of people, forced to watch pornography, forced to watch people having sex. Rape is when a man or boy forces a girl to have sexual intercourse with him. Sexual harassment includes threats of sexual attacks, demanding sex in exchange for something e.g. marks or job or a ride or accommodation. Other sexual harassment method are palm scratching, holding your hand or forcefully pulling and twisting your hand in such a way that it hurts. These can also happen to both boys and girls. Gender based violence results in, anxiety, depression low self-esteem and sexual difficulties. Gender based violence can make a person feel alone, worthless and scared.

Go back to the stories discussed at the beginning of this chapter, read them again. Try and identify which story is a good example of the following: physical abuse, emotional abuse, sexual abuse and sexual harassment.

The story of Ranisa is a good example of sexual abuse and it is called incest. Incest Is sexual activity between a child and a parent or between family members? Remember it is not right to experiment sexually with your family members. What has happened to Ranisa is sexual abuse and it is a criminal offence. This means that someone found guilty of this offence can go to jail

How can I help a friend who tells me that she/he has been abused?

- Listen
- Tell her/him that you believe what they have just said

- Support your friend
- Inform him/her of your legal obligation to report
- Refer him/her to a service in your community

Remember 8.1: It is not your fault that you are abused and you do not deserve it. Talk to someone you trust. You have a right to a life without abuse and you deserve it. Your body belongs to you no one else should be allowed to have control over it.

You have now finished your sexual health journey. You have probably reinforced the knowledge you already had about sexual health and probably learnt new things about sexual health and how to become sexually healthy. You have discovered who you are, how your body functions and how to live a healthy fulfilling life. Take a few minutes and think of all the positive things you do or have done in your life and congratulate yourself for this. Also think of the things you wish to improve on to ensure that you become sexually healthy and work on them. To conclude your journey on sexual health, try and answer this question "Are you sexually healthy?" I conclude this book with a summary of some of the statements made by participants in some of the sexual health workshops that I conducted.

I am sexually healthy because:

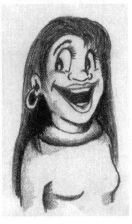

- I love myself.
- I love my body and understand how it functions.
- I think positively and feel good about myself and other.
- I feel wanted, accepted and cared for.

- I am courageous to face life with all its challenges.
- I take pride in my abilities, skills and accomplishments.
- I have better relationships with my family, teachers, peers and community.
- I treat my peers with respect and as equals.

- I do not discriminate against people because of their colour, location, nationality, tribe, sex and sexual orientation.
- I do not engage in practices that are harmful to others and me.
- I know how to say no to sex.
- I practice safer sex.

BIBLIOGRAPHY

Alberta Health and wellness (u.d) *Birth methods it's your choice*. Available: http://www.health.gov.ab.ca/public/bc-sx2.pdf.

Beels C, Hopson B & Scally M. 1988. Assertiveness: A positive process Leeds: Lifeskills

Canadian Health Network sexuality/Reproductive health. *Healthy living and promotion*. Available at www.ccohs.ca/headlines/sexsa.html.

Coetzee E, Hawksley H & Louw H. 2001. *Life Orientation today. Grade 9, Learner's book*. Cape Town: Maskew Miller Longman.

Cohen, YA. 1964. *The Transition from childhood to adolescence*. Chicago: Aldine Publishing Company.

Cornwall A & Welbourn A. 2002. *Realizing rights: Transforming approaches to sexual and reproductive well-being*. London: Zed Books

Crewe, M. 1996. Why is the subject of sex education for youth so difficult to deal with? A journey to honesty. *Sexual & reproductive health bulletin*, 3 September, 8-9.

Darroch, JE. Landry, DJ & Singh S. 2000 Changing emphases in sexuality education. *Family Planning Perspectives*, 32(5): 1-9.

De Miranda S. [Sa] *The South African Guide to Drugs and Drug Abuse*. Johannesburg: Michael Collins Publications cc

Delora JS & Warren CAB. 1977. *Understanding sexual interaction*. Boston: Houghton Miffin.

Fine, M. 1988. Sexuality, schooling and adolescent females: The missing discourse of desire. *Harvard Educational Review,* 58(1) February 1988: 29-53.

Galassi MD & Galassi JP. 1977. *Assert yourself: How to be your own person.* New York: Human Sciences Press.

Goosen, M. & Klugman, B. (editors). 1996. *The South African women's health book.* Cape Town: Oxford University Press.

Harrison D. 2002. *Lovelife campaign to encourage parents to "love them enough to talk about sex": rationale and results.* Johannesburg: Lovelife

HealthySA. 2003. Sexual Health Available: http//www.healthysa.sa.gov. au/

Hopson B & Scally M. 1980. *Lifeskills teaching programmes.* Leeds Lifeskills associates.

Hughes, H. 1994. Understanding sexual health. *Health Action,* 10 September-November: 4-5.

International family health. [Sa]. *Sexual health constituency.* International family health.

International Federation of Red Cross and Red Crescent Societies, [Sa]. *An introduction to sexual health.* International Federation of Red Cross and Red Crescent Societies.

Jakubowski, P & Lange, AJ. 1978. *The assertive option: Your rights and responsibilities.* Champaign, 111: Research Press Co

Koontz, S & Conly, SR. 1994. *Youth at risk: meeting the sexual health needs of adolescents - Questions and Answers. Population Action International,* April 1994.

Lindhard N & Dlamini N. 1990. *Lifeskills in the classroom.* Cape Town: Maskew Miller Longman

Lindhard N, Mathabe N & Atmore N. 1987. *Lifeskills in the communities: five teaching programmes.* Cape Town: University of Cape Town

Maluleke, T. 1997. Why do women have negative feelings about the first time they realised they were different from men. *Women's Health News,* November 24: 24-25.

National Guidelines Task Force, 1992. *Guidelines for comprehensive sexuality education.* Sex Information and Education Council of the U. S. New York

Rees, S & Graham RS. 1991. *Assertion training: how to be who you really are.* London: Routledge.

RHO. Gender and sexual health: Overview and lessons learnt. http://www.rho.org/html/gsh_overview.htm.

Roebuck C. 1998. Effective Communication. New York: McGraw-Hill.

Rooth E, Van der Straaten F, Maluleke T, Ferrira S & Mbhele E. 2008. OBE for FET colleges. Life orientation Level 4 Student's book. Cape Town: Nasou Via Africa. ISBN 978 1415402 092.

Rooth E, Van der Straaten F, Maluleke T, Ferrira S & Mbhele E. 2007. OBE for FET colleges. Life orientation Level 3 Student's book. Cape Town: Nasou Via Africa. ISBN 978 1415402 061.

Rooth E, Van der Straaten F, Maluleke T, Ferrira S & Mbhele E. 2007. OBE for FET colleges. Life orientation Level 2 Student's book. Cape Town: Nasou Via Africa. ISBN 978 1415402 030.

Rooth E, Van der Straaten F, Maluleke T, Ferrira S & Mbhele E. 2007. OBE for FET colleges. Life orientation Level 2 Lecturer's Guide. Cape Town: Nasou Via Africa. ISBN 978 141540 2054.

Rooth, E. 1995. *Lifeskills: A resource book for facilitators.* Cape Town: MacTIPS.

Sarrel LJ & Sarrel PM. 1979. Sexual unfolding: Sexual development and sex therapies in late adolescence. Boston: Little, Brown

Senderowitz, J. *Involving youth in reproductive health projects.* 1998. [Online] Available: Focus Web Site, http//www.pathfind.org/focus.htm

SIECUS. 1997. Adolescence and Abstinence Fact sheet. *SIECUS Report,* Vol 26(1) Available: http://www.siecus.org/pubs/fact/fact0001.html.

Smith MJ. 1975. *When I say no, I feel guilty: How to cope, using the skills of systematic assertive therapy.* New York: Bantam Books.

Spira A, Bajos N & the ACSF Group. 1994. *Sexual behaviour and AIDS.* Aldershot: Avebury.

Suekial R. 2002. *Being me, being you. Grade 6 Learner's book.* Cape Town: Kagiso Education.

Tannen, D. 1994. *Gender & discourse.* New York: Oxford University Press.

The Alan Guttmacher Institute. 2000.*Trends towards abstinence-only sex-ed means many U.S. Teenagers are not getting vital messages about contraception.* Available: New York News Release Web Site, http://www.agi-usa.org/ pubs/

Williams, S, Seed, J & Mwau, A. 1994. *The Oxfam gender training manual.* United Kingdom: Oxfam.

Thraves PA & Wilson, JS. 2002. *Finding and interpreting our worlds. Grade 6 Learner's book.* Lansdowne: ACE Publications

Townsend, A.1991. *Developing assertiveness.* London: Routledge.

UNICEF, AYA & PSI 2002 *Baseline study on knowledge, attitudes, behaviours and practices of adolescents and youth on sexual and reproductive health.* Botswana: UNICEF.

PART TWO

GET TO KNOW YOURSELF: A HANDBOOK FOR HEALTH PROMOTERS AND PEER EDUCATORS FACILITATING SEXUAL HEALTH AMONG YOUNG PEOPLE

Thelmah Xavela Maluleke

ABOUT THE HANDBOOK

"Get to know yourself: A handbook for health promoters and peer educators facilitating sexual health among young people" was developed mainly for health promoters and peer educators who facilitate sexual health education programmes in the community. The handbook must be used together with the "Get to know yourself: A sexual health guide for young people" book and all participants should have access to it especially during training. The handbook is meant for health promoters and young people who want to make a significant contribution towards the health and wellness of young people in their communities by becoming peer educators. They will use the handbook to facilitate peer educators workshops entitled "Get to know yourself: Sexual health education workshops" in their communities, churches, clubs, cultural organisations and traditional rites of passage. Although the main focus of the workshops is on young people, these workshops can also be used for more mature people to advance their knowledge on sexual health.

Sexual health peer educators who will use the handbook will be trained by health promoters, nurses, health educators, community health workers and others or can even train themselves by practicing facilitation as indicated in the handbook. The training runs over a period of one week, three days spent on the content and required skills, and practice over a period of two days for the peer educators to perfect facilitation skills. During the training sexual health peer educators will be guided on how to prepare and run the workshops effectively (**See aims of the peer educators training programme and competencies below).** It is advisable where possible, to allow peer educators/sexual health facilitators to conduct at least one workshop under the supervision of a health promoter/health educator/community health worker before conducting workshops on their own.

For effective training of peer educators, health promoters and self trained peer educators should use the "Get to know yourself: A handbook for health promoters and peer educators facilitating sexual health". This handbook will guide health promoters and peer educators in training peer educators and conducting sexual health education programmes in the communities. It is paramount that all participants attending the peer educators training have both books, "Get to know yourself: A sexual health guide for young people" and "Get to know yourself: A handbook for health promoters and peer educators facilitating sexual health". It is equally important that when conducting sexual health education workshops in the community that all participants have access to a copy of the "Get to know yourself: A sexual health guide for young people".

AIMS OF THE SEXUAL HEALTH PEER EDUCATORS TRAINING PROGRAMME

The aims of the sexual health peer educators training programme are:
- To train sexual health peer educators on facilitation skills, workshop planning, sexual health concepts, sexually transmitted infections and HIV and AIDS

- To train peer educators in creating a suitable environment in which peers can engage in open and honest discussion about sexuality and sexual health.
- To enable peer educators to use sexual health education principles in dealing with sexual health needs of young people as individuals and group.
- To enable sexual health peer educators to apply appropriate facilitation skills in the promotion of healthy sexual behaviours among young people in the communities.

CORE COMPETENCIES

On completion of the sexual health peer educators training programme, the peer educators must be competent in:

- Facilitating group discussions of sexual health topics among peers.
- Applying the peer education principles and skills to facilitate sexual health programmes among young people in the communities.
- Promoting sexual health and preventing risky sexual behaviours among young people, in the community.
- Mobilizing young people to initiate own sexual health, development and empowerment activities that promote healthy life styles
- Identifying sexual health learning needs of the individual and groups and develop strategies and use available technologies to deal with the identified learning in collaboration with other peer educators

- Planning and managing sexual health workshops and educational material resources to ensure that the aims of the sexual health workshops are successfully achieved.

To run the sexual health education workshops effectively, peer educators should also have the following skills which should have been acquired during their training:

- Democratic leadership and motivational skills
- Good communication skills which should be at the level of your peers
- Respect for peers and their views
- Ability to conduct discussions without personalizing the discussions
- Group management skills
- Facilitation skills

The handbook is divided into three parts, **Section one** reviews the meaning of peer education, key concepts related to sexual health and facilitation skills necessary to facilitate a sexual health workshop. **Section two** discusses preparations for the Get to know yourself: Sexual health education workshops. It provides information that will assist peer educators in planning and facilitating sexual health education programmes. It outlines the programme and activities that peer educators must use to facilitate sexual health education among their peers. **Section three** discusses the sexual health education workshop process including the activities and additional information that should be given to the participants.

SECTION 1: CONCEPT RELATED TO SEXUAL HEALTH PEER EDUCATION

What is sexual health?

Sexual health is defined as the integration of physical, emotional, intellectual and social aspects of sexual being in ways that are positively enriching, and that enhance personality, communication and love. It is the ability to have an informed, enjoyable, and safe sex life, based on a positive approach to sexual expression and mutual respect in sexual relations. In other words, sexual health means freedom from diseases, good relationship with yourself and others, and access to information that can enhance sexuality and relationships.

Sexual health acknowledges that human beings are sexual beings and have sexual rights. As sexual beings young people need to express and enjoy their sexuality throughout life and to take responsibility for their sexual behaviour. For you to exercise your sexual rights you need information, education, skills, support and services to make responsible decisions about your sexuality consistent with your own values. You need freedom from fear, shame, guilt, false beliefs and other factors that might inhibit your sexual response and impair your sexual relationship.

As a sexually healthy person you appreciate your body, take responsibility for your behaviour, and communicate with people in a respectful manner. You probably communicate respectfully with both females and males, young and old.

You also communicate effectively with family, peers and partners. You seek information to make informed choices, express love and intimacy consistent with your values in an appropriate way and you protect yourself from unwanted pregnancy, STIs and HIV/AIDS. In other words, a sexually healthy individual makes informed choices and does not engage in a sexual relationship that will later embarrass her or him. As a sexually healthy person you know your rights and you respect those of others. You are able to have a relationship that is non-exploitative and is based on shared values, honesty, and mutual pleasure

What is a health promoter?

The World Health Organisation defined health promotion as "the process of enabling people to increase control over, and to improve, their health. It moves beyond a focus on individual behaviour towards a wide range of social and environmental interventions". A health promoter is a health professional who work with communities and groups to plan and develop ways to help people improve and manage their health.

What is a health educator?

Health education is educating individuals, groups and communities about health, diseases, prevention of diseases and ways of keeping themselves healthy. Health educators work to encourage healthy lifestyles and wellness through educating individuals and communities about behaviours that promote healthy living and prevent diseases and other health problems. They communicate and advocate for health and health education. Health educators also serve as health education resource to patients by providing them with information to help prevent the problems associated with their conditions.

What is a community health worker?

A community health worker is trained member of community who has been selected in trust by his/her community to enter their homes and assist them to improve their health status. Community health workers reach out to the people and community groups at household and community level respectively. Their roles and activities are diverse within and across countries and across programmes. Community health workers perform a wide range of preventive, promotive, curative and/ or developmental programmes and interventions in the community and primary care facilities at community level. They communicate and advocate for health and health education and serve as health education resource to patients by providing them with information to help prevent the problems associated with their conditions.

What is peer education?

Peer education means sharing of valuable information among people of the same age group. The information in peer education is shared in a non-threatening democratic way. It needs people with democratic leadership skills to facilitate learning from each other among same age groups.

What is a peer educator?

A peer educator is a person who has some characteristics that are similar to those of the group she/he wants to facilitate. These characteristics could be age, colleagues at work, attending same school, grade, church, club including initiation ceremony.

What is sexual health peer education?

Sexual health peer education in this manual means sexual health education facilitated among young people by young people themselves. The sexual health education is based on the book entitled "Get to know yourself: A sexual health guide for young people" aimed at providing accurate information about sexual health that will enable young people to develop responsible sexuality, mutual respect between females and males, and good relationships that will result in the improvement of their quality of life.

Sexual health peer education is used in this programme to encourage sharing of information among young people with some acting as facilitators of discussions. It is a participatory method that involves young people in the discussion and activities. It empowers young people to take action against ignorance, poverty and diseases. It also empowers young people to take responsibility for their health and happiness.

Sexual health peer education takes place within a relaxed learning environment where young people feel free to ask questions on sexuality and are able to discuss without fear of being judged or labelled. It also gives young people an opportunity to discuss issues that are difficult to discuss with adults. Sexual health peer education encourages young people to gain insights through mutual sharing of experiences, knowledge and information.

Peer education means sharing of valuable information among people of the same age group. The information in peer education is shared in a democratic way. It needs people with democratic leadership skills to facilitate learning from each other among same age groups.

What is a sexual health peer educator?

Sexual health peer educators are young people trained to facilitate sexual health workshops among other young people. In other words a sexual health peer educator is a facilitator of a sexual health peer education programme in this case a sexual health peer educator is a peer educator who facilitates the **"Get to know yourself: Sexual health workshops"**. The sexual health peer educators help young people define their concerns and seek solutions through the mutual sharing of information and experiences. The sexual health peer educators must also disseminate new information and knowledge to the group members and become a role model by practicing what she/he teaches. She/he must be aware of where information and support for the peers can be found. Peer educators should also be sensitive, open minded, non-judgmental, trustworthy, good listeners and good communicators. She/he must be able to bring out the views and concerns of the peers and let young people make their own decisions based on facts. To be a good sexual health peer educator you need the following skills:

- Democratic leadership and motivation skills i.e. she/he must avoid being directive and authoritarian.
- Good communication skills which should be at the level of the peers. She/he must avoid paternalistic behaviours i.e. she/he must always remember that she/he is a peer not a parent
- Respect for your peers and their views
- Conduct discussions without personalizing the discussions
- Group management skills
- Group discussions management skills
- Facilitation skills

What are "Get to know yourself: sexual health workshops?
Get to know yourself: sexual health workshops" are workshops conducted among young people in groups of 20 participants facilitated by trained sexual health peer educators. At least two peer educators should facilitate each session.

The aims of these workshops are:

- To assist young people in understanding the human body;
- To assist young people to live a healthy fulfilling life with confidence and respect for themselves and others;
- To assist young people in gaining knowledge and skills that will enable them to form attitudes, beliefs and values about your body image, sexuality, development and interpersonal relationships;
- To assist young people in taking responsible steps to prevent teenage pregnancy, sexually transmitted infections (STI), HIV and AIDS.
- To assist young people in recognizing their role in their communities and as citizens of South Africa and the World.

The workshops will be conducted over a period of three days. The facilitation of the workshop will happen during plenary and small group sessions. Facilitation of a plenary session is done with all the participants and peer educators in one room. During small group discussion, participants will be divided in small groups of not more than six participants. Small groups are mainly used to encourage full participation by all the participants. During small group discussions, each group must choose a leader (who will lead the discussions) and a scriber who will be taking notes and present during plenary).

The reasons for using small groups and subgroups are the following:

- To ensure that young people benefit from knowledge and experiences of their peers
- To assist young people to examine their believes about other people

- To assist young people to collectively find new ways of looking at their own situation
- To encourage young people to accept each other's differences as basis for sharing experiences
- To develop the participants' confidence in expressing themselves
- To assist young people organize themselves and take responsibility for their situation

What is the role of a health promoter and peer educator/ facilitator in the sexual health workshops?

The main function of a health promoter and sexual health peer educators is to keep the group on track and encourage all the members to participate fully in all the discussions. These roles should be shared among the peer educators

- The facilitator must welcome and introduce the participants to one another through an activity
- Introduce the workshop aims
- Together with the participants develop ground rules
- Make sure the group agrees on, and works according to, the group rules
- Ask participants' their expectations and fears
- Match up expectations, aims and programme and make sure the group agrees on these.
- Encourage the participants to participate in the process and in decisions affecting the group
- Ensure that the group achieves the objectives of each session in the time available

- Give the group the necessary information, material e.g. flip chart, markers, or list of questions or activity that must be done in the small groups
- Keep the participants lively and active by using energizers when you see that their energy level is going down.
- At the end of each day, ask participant to answer the following questions: "What I learnt? What I have unlearnt? What I am taking with me?" and discuss their inputs.
- Evaluate the proceedings of the day
- Give them homework and make sure you get feedback on the homework every morning

In order to be effective, as a health promoter and sexual health peer educator you must have the ability to:

- Keep abreast of new information and knowledge in the area of sexual health.
- Listen and communicate effectively
- Deal with emotions and difficult situation
- Be non-judgemental attitude and ability to express emotions
- Be adaptive and flexible nature
- Encourage and provide support
- Lead by example
- Maintain confidentiality information and trust
- Look at things from various perspectives
- Make decisions and encourage others to do so.
- Facilitate learning among young people in your community
- Manage time efficiently
- Be assertive
- Plan and run sexual health workshops properly

- Conduct all activities properly
- Use energizers to keep the group awake, attentive and lively/ also encourage participants to come up with energizers when the need arises.

What is facilitation?

Facilitation means enabling groups to learn in an environment that allows them to participate as equals. Facilitation ensures that the group achieves its goals and objectives and encourages active participation from everyone.

What is a facilitator?

A facilitator is an individual who enables groups to work more effectively and collaborate to achieve set goals/objectives. It is someone who skillfully helps a group of people understand their common objectives and assist them to plan to achieve them without taking sides in the discussion.

What a sexual health peer educator should not do.

A good sexual health peer educators should not:

- Downplay people's ideas
- Push personal agendas and opinions
- Dominate the group
- Continuously read from the notes
- Tell inappropriate offensive stories or lie to the group
- Allow people to bully others
- Taking sides during discussion
- Tell too much about their personal experiences and life
- Back a particular opinion

- Let the group to unconsciously or consciously shy away from a difficult area of sexual health
- Lead the group towards what she/he thinks is the right direction

SECTION TWO: PREPARATION FOR THE GET TO KNOW YOURSELF: SEXUAL HEALTH WORKSHOP

Planning for the workshop

The sexual health workshop facilitated by peer educators runs over a period of three to five days. It is facilitated by four facilitators. Before you can run a workshop you need to plan as a team of peer educators in your village. Planning is important because it determines the success of your workshop. A well planned workshop is good for the facilitators, participant and success of the programme. Your workshop plan should try and answer the following questions:

- What do we want to achieve? Describe the aims/purpose of the workshops.
- Who are the facilitators and how are they going to be involved? Allocate tasks to all the facilitators and share the tasks and responsibilities
- Who are the participants? Decide on the number of participants, how you will recruit them? How are they going to be registered? Are they going to pay registration fee? How much is the registration fee?
- Where is the workshop going to be conducted? Inform the relevant authorities about the workshop. Get permission to run the workshop where necessary. Organise and book a suitable venue with chairs that can be moved around.

- What equipment do you need for the workshop?
  Organise name & desktop tags, flip charts, press-stik, marking pens, participants' files, pens, writing pads, copies of the programme, camera or photographer,

- What refreshments and meals are going to serve? Who will supply the refreshments? Who will prepare and serve the refreshments? Make sure you have an independent person or company to prepare the meals and refreshments.

- When is the workshop going to be conducted? Decide on whether you are going to run the workshop during the week or on weekends. Decide on the duration of the workshop and each session of the workshop.

- How is the programme going to look like? Draw the workshop programme with all the sexual peer educators who are going to be facilitator. Allocate roles for each facilitator including the time keeper. Decide on a time for mock workshop to practice the allocated roles. Make sure that each facilitator will perform their role as required and facilitate their sessions well.

- Confirm attendance of the workshop with all your participants. Ask participants to bring along pictures of themselves (if they have them) at different stages of their development.

- The programme below is a guide feel free to use as is or adjust it to suit the needs of your participants

Draw a programme for the workshop

The programme below is an example that can be used for developing the sexual health workshops programme you intend facilitating.

Sample workshop programme

Topic	Session	Time allocation
Day 1		
Welcome & Introductions to the workshop and aims of the workshop	1	08:00
Introduction of participants and facilitators	2	08h15
Setting of ground rules	3	09h15
Expectations, fears and participants contribution to the success of the workshop	4	09h30
Pre-test	5	10h15
Tea		
Who am I?	5	10h30
Building self concept	6	11h30
Assertive skills	7	12h30
Lunch		
What does my body look like?	8	13h30
Human developmental stages	9	14h30
Summary & evaluation of the day's proceedings	10	15h45
Closure		**16h00**
Day 2		
What are relationships?	11	08h00
How do I keep myself healthy?	12	09h00

Tea		
I am a virgin?	13	10h30
I am sexually active What are the consequences of being sexually active?	14	11h30
What infections or diseases can I get if I am sexually active?	15	12h30
Lunch		
What is HIV and AIDS	16	13h30
Summary & evaluation of the day's proceedings	17	15h45
Closure		**16h00**

Day 3		
What cancers can affect the reproductive systems (male & female)	18	08h00
Tea		
What is gender based violence?	19	10h30
Lunch		
What is my role and responsibility as a young person in this community	19	13h00
Summary of the workshop	22	14h30
Evaluation	23	15h00
Closure		**15h30**

SECTION 3: THE SEXUAL HEALTH WORKSHOP PROCESS

Write down the objectives of the day on a flip chart before the workshop begins. Go through the objectives with the participants. At the end post the objectives on the wall.

DAY 1: DEVELOPING THE EMOTIONAL AND PSYCHOLOGICAL COMPONENT OF BEING

Objectives of the day (What must be achieved today?)

At the end of the day my peers should be able to:
- Remember each other names and address each other by name
- Appreciate who they are and feel good about themselves
- Relate well to their emotional and psychological component of their being
- Display and relate comfortably with self and develop good self concept
- Apply assertive skills in their daily lives
- Describe the functions of some parts of their bodies

Session 1: Welcome & Introductions to the workshop and aims of the workshop

During this session welcome your participants and show your appreciation for their attendance. Give a brief explanation of the workshop and its aims. Allow them to ask questions regarding the workshop. Briefly describe the objectives of the day

Session 2: Introduction of participants and facilitators

During this session participants and facilitators must introduce themselves to the group. There are many methods or exercises that can be used to facilitate introductions. You can also come up with innovative ways for the introductions. After they have introduced themselves issue out name tags if you have not given them out already during registration. Ask them to write down the names that they want the group to use during the workshop. Names are important because participants should always be addressed by their names.

Session 3: Setting of ground rules

With your participants set ground rules for your workshop. Ask each participant to mention one ground rule that they think is important for the smooth running of the workshop. List the ground rules on a flip chart and paste them on the wall.

Session 4: Expectations, fears and participants contribution to the success of the workshop

Activity 1

Ask each participant to give one expectation, one fear and her/his contribution to the success of the workshop. List these on three separate flip charts marked as follows: flip chart number one, "Expectation", number two "Fears" and the last one "My contributions to the success of the workshop". List the participants' contributions accordingly. After the lists are complete, paste all the flip charts on the wall. Together with the participants, go through the list of expectation. Then unveil the objectives of the workshop objectives and compare with their expectation to find out if their expectations will be covered by the objectives of the workshop. Address each fear listed on the flip chart. Then address all the contributions listed.

Revisit the objectives of the day

Bring the flip chart with the objectives of the day to the fore and take the participants through them again. Paste them on the wall and inform your participants that the objectives will be revisited at the end of the day to find out if the objectives have been achieved.

Energizer

Conclude this activity with an energizer that promotes mingling, laughter and encouraging using and remembering the participants' names.

Session 5: Knowledge of participants regarding sexual health

Conduct a pretest

Introduce the pretest and its purpose. Inform them that it is an individual test and that it should not be discussed with their friends. Distribute the pretest and allow them 30 minutes to complete the test. Ask participants to put the pretest in a closing folder or envelope. When all the tests are submitted seal the file or envelop and put away. Do not look or read the answered tests in front of them.

Session 6: Who am I?

The question "Who am I?" requires a person to identify her/himself from others. It requires you to define yourself as you see yourself. I therefore want us to do an exercise that will define us from others.

Activity 2

Do exercise 1 from the book "Get to know yourself: A sexual health guide for young people". Allow each participant to present her/his answers to the questions. There will be a lot of emotions attached to their presentation. You must be ready to comfort these who are emotional. Then summarise the activity by reading out the statements under Remember 1.1.

Session 7: Building self concept

Introduce this session by reading the passage below to the participants.

"A person is a physical being (biological composition), emotional being (self-concept), social being (relationships) and sexual being and that sexual health is the integration of the physical, emotional and social aspects of the person's sexual being. Your emotional being can affect your physical being, social being and sexual being. The same is true of your social being: it can affect how you see yourself, feel about yourself and your sexual behaviour. What is good about this relationship is that if you improve your emotional being (self-concept) you can improve all the others. In other words, building your self-concept is the key to improving your wellbeing, including sexual health. Since the self-concept is the main key to our lives, our discussion will start with the emotional being and progress to the physical being and lastly the social being."

What can I do to build my self-concept?

To build your self-concept you need to develop skills to make you feel good about yourself. You have to strengthen your communication and assertive skills. You also need to develop those social skills that enable you to negotiate throughout your life. In other words we need to feel good about ourselves, we need to communicate clearly and in an assertive way, and we need to build positive relationships with our sisters, brothers, parents, grandparents, relatives, friends, teacher and community

Activity 3

Give each participant a sheet of paper with two columns. "Labels given to me" and "what I am". Ask participants to write down negative or bad labels given them by themselves and others. On the other column they must write the opposite of what is written on the left. They must try and remember all the positive things that their families and others have said about them. When they have finished writing ask them to cut the paper along the dividing line. Have a bowl or tin with water ready. Ask the participants to take the left side of the paper and say "This is not who I am" and put the paper in the water and wash it until it is in small particles. As they wash it off they must continue saying "This is not who I am". Tell each one of them that they have now removed all the negative labels. It is up to them not to allow the negative labels come back.

Why is it important to remove negative labels?

Negative labels destroy your confidence and make you feel bad about yourself.

These types of feelings can stop us from making friends or performing well at school. It is important to rid ourselves from of these labels and the change start with each one of us. We must stop dishing out negative labels to our brothers, sisters, parents, disabled people, friends and other people in our community. We must stop giving negative names to ourselves and others. Before you sleep every night take a count of bad things you said to yourself or to others. Say to yourself "I will always say good things to myself and other" repeat this statement several times.

Ask the participants to take the papers with "what I am" and duplicate if they want and put them in places where they will be able to read them. For example, next to the mirror, in their purse, school bags etc. Conclude by saying, "It is our responsibility and our right to love and believe in ourselves and we can do it".

Summary

To summarise the discussion use the bulleted statements under "This is what you do to claim back your self-concept:". Write the statements on small papers and ask participant to pick one and read aloud with some demonstration/acting out what the statement means with vigour and conviction. Prepare the small papers before the workshop.

Session 8: Assertive skills

There are three ways in which we might respond when situations arise in our lives. These responses are assertiveness (assertive behaviour), non-assertiveness (non-assertive behaviour) and aggressiveness (aggressive behaviour). Have the definitions of these concepts on a flip chart before the session. Unveil one definition at a time and discuss it with participants. Ask participants to give examples of each as you go through them.

What is being assertive?

It is an honest and appropriate expression of one's feelings, opinions, and needs. It also means communicating what you really want in a clear fashion, respecting your own rights and feelings and the rights and feelings of others. It is standing up for your rights and not being taken advantage of.

What is assertive behavior?

Assertive behavior is behavior that enables a person to act in his own best interests, to stand up for himself without undue anxiety, to express his honest feeling comfortably, or to exercise his own rights without denying the rights of others.

What is assertiveness?

Assertiveness is the direct and honest expression and communication of your thoughts, opinions, wishes, feelings, needs, and rights in a way that does not violate the personal rights of others. It involves standing up for your own rights, while acknowledging the rights of others, and working towards a win-win solution. In other words, assertiveness is standing up for your right to be treated fairly.

Assertiveness includes:

- Starting, changing, or ending conversations
- Sharing feelings, opinions, and experiences with others
- Making requests and asking for favors
- Refusing others' requests if they are too demanding
- Questioning rules or traditions that don't make sense or don't seem fair
- Addressing problems or things that bother you
- Being firm so that your rights are respected
- Expressing positive emotions
- Expressing negative emotions

Assertiveness is different from non-assertiveness and aggressiveness. People who are not aware of the difference often use aggression thinking that they are being assertive or become submissive thinking that they are assertive.

What is non-assertiveness?

Non-assertiveness (or submissiveness) is when you allow others to violate your rights by regarding their needs, opinions and rights as more important than your own. This shows a lack of respect for your own needs and can lead to feelings of hurt, anxiety and anger.

What is aggressiveness?

Aggressiveness is the opposite of non-assertiveness. It involves expressing and pursuing your rights at the expense of others, which creates the impression of disrespect for the other person. In effect, you are getting your own way, no matter what other people think. This, in turn, can lead to people having less respect for you.

Activity 4

Divide the participants in pairs and ask them to do Exercise 2: Assertive skills from the "Get to know yourself: Sexual health guide for young people". Firstly, they must indicate how they would have responded to the situation and why? Secondly, ask them to indicate the type of responses displayed by James, Langa and Larry and why? Ask each group to report back. Write their feedback on the flip chart.

Conclude this activity by stating the following:

When we are assertive we tell a person what we want, or need or would prefer. We state this clearly and confidently. We stand up for our rights; express honest personal rights without denying the rights of others. We show respect to ourselves and others. We develop caring honest relationship with others. We have the ability to ask for support when we need it. We promote equality in human relationships. Assertive behaviour enables us to act in our best interests, to stand up for ourselves without anxiety. It builds our self-confidence.

How can being non-assertive affect my life/academic performance?

When you behave or interact in a non-assertive manner, you allow your own needs to go unmet. There are many ways in which this could be harmful to your life to your academic life. One of the most common occurs when you allow family or friends to take up time you had set aside for task you must perform or study. For instance, if you have an assignment or homework or chores due tomorrow and your friends ask you to go out with them tonight, a person who was non-assertive might feel unable to say 'no', and would end up going out instead of doing the assignment, homework or chores. Another way non-assertiveness can affect your academic life would be when you believe, correctly, that you deserved more marks for an assignment, but take the non-assertive approach of doing nothing about it. This could make the difference between passing or failing the course overall. Finally, not asking for clarification of a point your teachers has made and that you do not understand can also be considered non-assertiveness. This could mean you miss out on some information that is vital for the exam.

Session 9: What does my body look like?

Every day we bath our bodies and apply some lotions and oils to them, but we do not have time to touch and feel our bodies mainly because we are in hurry. I want us to spend time with our bodies.

Activity 5

Introduce this activity by saying: Let us all stand up and move our chairs backwards to give ourselves some room. Let us make sure that we have enough space to stretch our hands without touching the people next to us. I want all of us to close our eyes and follow my instructions.

Close your eyes. Take a deep slow breath and fill your lungs with air. Slowly allow the air to escape through your nose and mouth. Again, take a deep slow breath and fill your lungs with air. Slowly allow the air to escape through your nose and mouth. Relax. Using both hands, slowly touch your head, feel the circumference of your head and the texture of your hair. Stroke your hair backwards and feel it. If you have no hair just feel your hand as you brush your scalp. Slowly move your hand to your fore head feel it.

Move your hands to your eyebrows feel the eyebrows. Then move your hands to your closed eyes feel your eyes moving. Then feel your nose, your mouth and cheeks. Touch your neck feel it. Move your hands around your neck. Move your hands down to your chest, abdomen and back. Touch each part with love and care.

Feel your hands as they move down your body. Touch your arms, elbows and fingers feel them. Slowly move down your body to your legs, knees, ankles and toes. Feel them as you touch them. Feel how your body accepts the attention and love that you have just given it. Slowly open your eyes. We have completed our exercise. How do you feel? We need to touch our bodies with feelings every time. When we have a bath consciously wash it with love and care. Feel all the parts as you touch them. We need to know our bodies and have an everlasting friendship with it. We also need to know and understand how the different parts of our bodies function.

The human body

Exercise 3

In plenary ask for volunteers to read and act out the story about Stomach pains from the "Get to know yourself: A sexual health guide for young people".

Conclude this exercise by indicating that:

The human body consists of different systems that work together to form a whole. The body functions like a machine, car or bicycle. The different parts should work together in order for it to function properly. The body functions in the same way. When you look at yourself you just see one person, but inside you there are ten systems working very hard to keep you alive. You do not hear or feel the systems working unless there is a problem.

Activity 6

In groups of four discuss the following systems:
- Group 1: skin, muscular and skeletal system
- Group 2: circulatory and Lymphatic system
- Group 3: respiratory and digestive system
- Group 4: urinary, endocrine and nervous system

In your groups discuss the allocated system according to the following headings:
- List the parts that form the system allocated to you.
- What is the function of each part or system in the body?
- What will happen if this system is not working properly or stops working completely?
- What do we need to do to ensure that this system functions as required?

Each group gives a feedback at plenary. Encourage them to go and read more about their bodies.

Conclude this activity by asking the participants to do **Activity 7**

Activity 7
Ask the participants to take a few minutes and think about the questions below:

- Why is it important to understand the human body and how it functions?
- Why is it important to keep our bodies clean at all times?
- How are you going to use the information about our bodies in your own life?
- What are you going to do to ensure that your friends learn about their bodies?

In their groups they must discuss their answers to the questions and present their answers in plenary. Write the answers on a flip chart and paste on the wall.

The reproductive system
The reproductive system is the system that is responsible for procreation and multiplication of people in the world. Females and males have different reproductive organs, often referred to as sex organs.

Activity 8
In groups of four people of female and male only participants, ask the female and male only groups to discuss the female reproductive organs and male groups respectively in their separate groups. Bring the groups to plenary discuss the female and male organs using the diagrams in the

"Get to know yourself: A sexual health guide for young people". Encourage participants to ask questions and to use the names of the reproductive parts without feeling uncomfortable or embarrassed. At the end of the discussion ask the following questions:

Ask participants how they felt when they discussed the reproductive systems in small groups of the same sex?

Ask participants how they felt when the male and female reproductive organs were discussed in plenary?

Address their feelings accordingly.

Ask the participants how they feel now?

Encourage participants to feel comfortable in discussing reproductive organs with peers and mixed group of participants.

In conclusion read "Remember 2.3 from the "Get to know yourself: Sexual health guide for young people".

Session 10: Summary and evaluation of the day

Summarise the day by revisiting the objectives. Go through each objective and ask the participants if the objective has been achieved. Ask the participants individually to give one of the activities of the day they remember.

Evaluation of the day

To evaluate the day put the following questions and statement on a flip chart: "What have I learnt?" "What have I unlearned?" "The message I am taking with me" Ask each participant to give an answer for each question and statement. Write their answers on a flip chart. Paste it on the wall.

DAY 2: HUMAN DEVELOPMENTAL STAGES AND HEALTHY LIVING

Objectives of the day (What must be achieved today?)

At the end of the day the participants/ my peers should be able to:

- Appreciate and understanding developmental stages they are experiencing or have experienced
- Assist and guide other young people experiencing developmental changes and challenges to understand the changes that are happening in their body
- Have healthy relationships with self, family, peers and partners
- Take responsibility and communicate with people (males and females) in a respectful manner.
- Take responsibility to seek information and prevent the spread of STIs, HIV and AIDS
- Develop positive ways of dealing with challenges in their lives and still maintain healthy lives.

Session 11: Human Developmental stages

Activity 10

Ask participants to do Exercise 4 from the "Get to know yourself: Sexual health guide for young people" book. Take a few minutes to think about yourself when you were still a child and the different stages you have gone through until now. What changes do you see? Then discuss the different stages and changes that occur from infancy to adulthood.

Activity 11

In groups of four people, female and male only participants, ask the female only groups to read "The story of Margaret" and male only groups to read the "The story of George". Give each group a sheets of paper to answer the questions below:

- What is the story all about?
- Does it happen in real life situation?
- What can you do to deal with the situation?
- What are you going to do to ensure that this does not happen to other young people?

Allow the groups present in plenary. Discuss issues that are brought up in details.

Give more information

Discuss the menstrual cycle and wet dreams and erections among boys during puberty in details.

Conclude the discussions by reading "Remember 2.3, 2.4, 2.5 and 2.6"

Conclude by asking for four volunteers to read one stanza each from the poem entitled... "I love you my body" from the "Get to know yourself: A sexual health guide for young people" book

Session 12: What are relationships?

Activity 12

In plenary ask participants what they understand by relationships. Write their views on a flip chart. Go through the list and discuss each one of them.

Activity 13

Ask the participants to close their eyes. Take them through this in a nice calm and clear voice.

"Close your eyes and imagine yourself walking alone down a beautiful path. As you walk down you feel calm and at ease with yourself. You walk down the descending road until you reach a beautiful gate. Someone, an adult you know and trusts joins you at the gate. Quietly you both walk down slowly through the gate. Who is this person? As you slowly walk down you decide to sit down under a beautiful tree and enjoy its shade. Your companion quietly sits beside you and smile. You then notice some movements at a distance. It's a child, slowly walking towards you. As the child approaches, you notice some resemblance. The child looks like you! You look at the child again wanting to get some sense of the child's feelings. Is the child happy? Why? Is the child sad? Why? There are many questions that are racing through your mind as you look at the child. You realize that it is getting late you start moving back with your companion. As you walk back you realize that the child is also walking besides you. As you walk towards the gate you realise that you are actually holding each other's hands. When you get to the gate your adult companion says to you 'THE CHILD NEXT TO YOU IS YOU. LOVE AND RESPECT YOURSELF. FEEL GOOD ABOUT YOURSELF AND ALWAYS LIVE AND THINK POSITIVELY'. Slowly open your eyes. Stretch yourself and shake your body. How do you feel?

Activity 14

Divide participants into groups of five to discuss the questions:

• How did you feel as you were walking towards the gate without the companion?

- How did you feel after you were joined by the adult?
- Who was the adult who accompanied you?
- What is your relationship with the adult who was walking with you?
- How was the child? Did the child look happy? Why? or Did the child look sad? Why?
- You were told to love and respect yourself. What does it mean to you?
- You were also told to feel good about yourself and always think positively? What does it mean to you?
- Allow the participants to present their answers to the questions and discuss their answers thoroughly and give more information about relationships.

What skills do I need in order to have good relationships?

Activity 15

Allow the participants to give their own views and write the responses on a flip chart. Then ask for volunteers (one statement per volunteer) to read the statements under the heading, "What skills do I need in order to have good relationships?" from the "Get to know yourself: A sexual health guide for young people" book.

How do I maintain a good relationship with my family?

Allow the participants to give their own views and write the on a flip chart. Then take their contribution and add more information where necessary.

How to have a trusting relationship with your family?

Activity 16

Allow the participants to give their own views and write the on a flip chart. Then take them through the statements below: Read the bulleted statements or ask the participants to read the statements or you can write then in small papers and give them to participants to read out).

If you want your family to trust you:

- You have to be truthful.
- When you talk to your parents be clear and specific about what you are saying.
- Also ensure that your family is aware of your feelings about what is happening within the family.
- Express your appreciation and affection to your family members.
- Develop and maintain a positive relationship with your sisters and brothers. Encourage mutual support during family crises.
- Show your parents that you are responsible by keeping your promises and facing the consequences of your actions.
- Know your rights and ensure that they are not violated.
- Another important thing in your relationship with your parents is to ask for forgiveness if you have wronged them and to forgive them if they make mistakes.

How do I maintain a good relationship with my friends?

Activity 17

Allow the participants to give their own views and write the on a flip chart. Take them through the information they have given. Give additional information on good relationships with friends. Conclude this activity by indicating that:

- Good or positive relationships are those that are supportive, helpful and lead to happy interactions.
- Helpful relationships are those that support your goals, values, needs and interests.
- Good relationships are marked by good communication and understanding, as well as respect for each other.
- Good relationships have boundaries that should not be crossed.

'Write the statements below on small papers and ask participants to pick one paper and read aloud and act out what the statement depicts where possible.'

Good friends are **HONEST**.
They communicate openly and truthfully. They admit their mistakes. They say how they feel. They don't tell lies to each other.

Good friends **PROMOTE EQUALITY**
Friends ensure that the relationship is equal. There is no one in charge or giving orders to others. There is no one person who is more important than another.

Good friends are **LOYAL**
They do not gossip about each other, or end friendships for no reason.

Good friends **LAUGH TOGETHER**
They share jokes and have fun. Make you feel safe. They don't make you take risks, put you in danger or hurt you.

Good friends are **TOLERANT**
They forgive each other. They allow each other to make mistakes. They are patient, understanding and accepting.

Good friends are **FAIR**. They are able to compromise. They look for satisfying solution to conflict. Their negotiations are fair and democratic.

Good friends **SUPPORT EACH OTHER**.
They give each other help, encouragement, comfort and acceptance. They support each other's life goals.

Good friends are **INCLUSIVE.**

They accept you for who you are.

Good friends **SHARE**. Friends tell each other things. They share ideas, joys and tragedies. They are also willing to share resources and belongings.

Good friends **ACCEPT EACH OTHER**.

They don't want to change you to suit their needs.

Good friends **SHOW RESPECT FOR EACH OTHER.**

They listen to one another. They value each other's views. They do not judge. They understand affirm or encourage each other. They respect each other's right to their own feelings, interests and opinions.

Good friends are **TRUSTWORTHY.**

Friends are able to speak in confidence to each other. They know that their secrets will be safe.

Good friends accept friendship **BOUNDARIES**

Friends tell each other their set boundaries. They know that their friends respect their set boundaries. They do not allow their friends to overstep their boundaries. They know that if a friend is overstepping their boundaries it means their relationship is not healthy or good.

Boundaries in relationship

Relationships have boundaries. We should not allow people to overstep the boundaries we have set. If someone is overstepping your boundaries it means the relationship is not healthy or good.

Activity 18

Ask for a volunteer to read the statement under crossing or overstepping boundaries

Crossing or overstepping boundaries

If people do the following, they may be overstepping your boundaries meaning that the relationship is not healthy or good:

- Touching you without your permission.
- Swearing and shouting at you calling you names.
- Shaming and ridiculing you.
- Giving you orders at work in a rude and disrespectful way.
- Taking your personal belonging without asking.
- Listening to your personal conversations or phone messages and spreading your SMSs, e-mails or letters your consent.
- Sending abusive tweets and facebook posting about you.
- Exposing you to physical illness or danger.
- Not negotiating when, where and how to engage in sex.
- Demanding unsafe sexual practices.

If you do any of these things, you will also overstep other people's boundaries.

Adapted from **the FET colleges Life orientation Level 2** *page* **25.**

Conclude by saying:

Healthy relationships are those in which the rights of each individual are valued and respected. They are relationships based on equality, not on power and control. In healthy relationship, each person has rights.

Session 13: How do I keep myself healthy?

The concept "health" has been defined as a state of complete wellbeing that is physical, mental, social and spiritual. It does not only mean the absence of diseases or infirmity. To be healthy in this context means you have no physical, mental, emotional or social problems, of which it is impossible. To be healthy you need to build a good relationship with yourself, your family, your teachers, colleagues, your friends and elders in your community. Being healthy means you have self-esteem and good relationships with yourself, family, partner and community. To have self-esteem you need to love yourself and believe in yourself. Take control of your life and live positively.

What does positive living mean?

Activity 19

Allow the participants to give their own views and write them on a flip chart. Then take them through the information they provided and add where appropriate. Take them through the following paragraphs.

Although the 'phrase' positive living is as old as the human beings themselves, this phrase became more popular with the intensification of the HIV and AIDS epidemic. Positive living comes from the understanding that a person has the physical (the body), emotional (self-concept) and spiritual components which are linked together and any change in one can have profound effects on the other two. For example, physical aches and pains can make a person to become irritable and refuse to associate with other people (isolate) and even stop believing in her/his religion. Stress can lead to physical and spiritual imbalances. Emotional and physical illnesses can also be caused by spiritual imbalances.

Positive living is about maintaining a balance even when one or more of the human components are affected. It means living a healthy life even when a person is living with a chronic condition or disease. Positive living encourages a person to make the most of what remains of her/his when she/he has a physically or emotionally or spiritually imbalance. Positive living helps an individual to live a stress free life, maintain good physical and emotional health. It requires us as human being to understand that in our daily lives there are many things that can affect our physical, emotional and spiritual well being and we need to develop a positive ways of dealing with all these challenges and still maintain our equilibrium and healthy life.

How do I keep myself healthy?

Activity 20

Allow the participants to give their own views and write their views on a flip chart. Then take them through the information below:

Health means different things to different people and therefore, being healthy also means different things to different people. What does being healthy mean to you? How do you consider yourself healthy or not healthy, and why? If you consider yourself healthy, what do you need to do to remain healthy? If you consider yourself unhealthy, what do you need to do to be healthy? Discuss in twos. Ask participants to report on what their partners contributions. Write on the flip chart and discuss.

What I need to do in order to be healthy or remain healthy?

Activity 21

Allow the participants to give their own views and write them on a flip chart. Then ask for volunteers to read the statements 1 to 11 under "What does being healthy mean?" from the "Get to know yourself: A sexual health guide for young people".

What can I do to keep my environment clean and safe?

Activity 22

Allow the participants to give their own views and write the on a flip chart. Ask the participants to go out and assess the environment surrounding the workshop venue. When they return ask them to discuss their observation in groups. Depending on their findings ask them to answer one of the following questions:

What can we do to keep our environment clean? or What can we do to maintain a clean environment at all times?

What type of food must I eat to keep myself healthy?

Activity 23

Ask each participant to record the food they ate in the past 3 days. Ask each participant to present their list. Record the foods and tally as they present from the most eaten to least eaten foods. Rank the foods in order of preference from the tallies made.

Ask participants (in groups) to classify the foods they have listed according to the type of nutrients found in them e.g. carbohydrates (starch), protein, fibre, fat and vitamins. Allow each group to present their classification. Go through each list and correct where necessary.

How do exercises contribute to my health?

Activity 24

Ask participants (in groups) to give their views on how exercises contribute to their health and write their answers on the flip chart. What sporting or recreational activities are they involved in? What sporting codes and facilities are available in their community? What recreational activities and facilities are available in their community? What needs to be done to encourage young people to participate in sport and recreational activities? Allow each group to present their answers and discuss the answers with the participants.

What harmful practices must I avoid?

Activity 25

Ask participants (in groups) to list the harmful practices that young people engage in. Allow each group to present their list and record their presentation on a flip chart. Go through list and ask them why the practice is harmful? What can be done to prevent young people from becoming the victims of each harmful practice?

What is substance abuse?

Activity 26

Ask participants to give their view of what substance abuse is about and write their answers on the flip chart. Ask to list the common substances that are abused in their community. Ask them to give signs that will make them suspect that their friend or sibling is abusing drugs or alcohol. What steps will they take to assist a person who is abusing alcohol or drugs?

Conclude this session by reading "Remember 4.1 and 4.2" from the "Get to know yourself: A sexual health guide for young people" book.

Session 14: I am a virgin

Activity 27

What is a virgin?

Allow the participants to give their own views and write the on a flip chart.

Then take them through the information below:

A virgin is a male or female who has never had penetrative sex or sexual intercourse. You can have a relationship but choose not to have penetrative sex with your partner.

Exercise 5

Ask participants to read the story of John and Martin from the "Get to know yourself: A sexual health guide for young people" book and answer the questions following the story. Go through their answers and add more information on virginity for both males and females.

Conclude by reading "Remember 5.1 and 5.2".

Session 15: I am sexually active

Exercise 7

Ask participants to read Joyce's story from the "Get to know yourself: A sexual health guide for young people" and answer the questions below it. Give them flip charts to write and present their answers to the questions.

Conclude by reading "Remember 6.1".

What are the consequences of being sexually active?

Activity 28

Allow the participants to give their own views and write the on a flip chart and present. Then take them through the Exercise 8 from the "Get to know yourself: A sexual health guide for young people" book. Ask them to write their answers on flip charts and present in plenary. Discuss their answers in details and add where necessary. Include contraception in your discussion.

In conclusion:

Read Remember 6.2 and 6.3.

Session 16: What are sexually transmitted infections?

Ask participants to give their own views regarding STIs and write them on a flip chart. Then take them through the information they provided and add more information on STIs:

Exercise 9

Ask participants in groups to read the story "I am not feeling very well" from the Get to know yourself: Sexual health guide for young people" book and answer the following questions:

- What is wrong with Maggie?
- What must she do to deal with her problem?
- What are the signs of sexually transmitted infections
- What must you do if you suspect that you could be having STIs
- How can one protect her/himself from sexually transmitted infections?

Discuss their answers and add signs of STIs and how they can protect themselves from STIs

Session 17: Summary and evaluation of the day

Summarise the day by revisiting the objectives. Go through each objective and ask the participants if the objective has been achieved. Ask the participants individually to give one of the activities of the day they remember.

Evaluation of the day

To evaluate the day put the following on a flip chart: "What have I learnt?" "What have I unlearned?" "The message I am taking with me" Ask each participant to give an answer for each question and statement. Write their answers on a flip chart. Paste it on the wall.

DAY 3: DISEASE PREVENTION AND MY ROLE AND RESPONSIBILITIES

Objectives of the day (What must be achieved today?)

At the end of the day the participants should be able to:

- Take the necessary steps support people who are infected and affected by HIV and AIDS
- Take the necessary steps to prevent cancers that affect the reproductive system and encourage early detection and treatment of these cancers
- Take the necessary steps to prevent gender discrimination and gender-based violence
- Commit themselves to taking care of their own physical, spiritual and social wellbeing at all times and live healthy fulfilling lives
- Commit themselves to dealing with sexual health challenges that young people face in their communities, South Africa and globally.

Session 18: What are HIV and AIDS?

Ask the participants to give their own views about HIV and AIDS and write them on a flip chart. Then give them information on the HIV and AIDS and its effects worldwide and in your own country.

Activity 29

In groups ask participants to discuss the following questions and present their answers in plenary.

- What are HIV and AIDS?
- How is HIV passed from one person to another?
- How can I protect myself against HIV and AIDS?
- How do I know that I am living with HIV?
- If I am HIV positive what do I need to do to live longer?
- What can we do as young people to support those that are sick because of HIV and AIDS?
- What can we do as young people to support young people who are orphaned because of HIV and AIDS?
- What community support structures are available for HIV infected and affected persons?
- What is the government doing to prevent the spread of HIV
- What is the government doing to support those that are infected and affected by HIV and AIDS
- In your view what else should the government and community to support those that are infected and affected by HIV and AIDS

Go through the presentations and identify issues that need to be clarified and explain in details.

Activity 30

What does positive living mean in the context of HIV and AIDS or any illness? Allow the participants to give their own views and write them on a flip chart. Go through the presentations and identify issues that need to be clarified and explain in details.

Then go through the information below:

There is as yet no cure for HIV and AIDS. However a lot is known on how to avoid transmission of the virus to others and how to prevent becoming infected yourself. Living positive with HIV is when a person has accepted the condition and allow her/his family to give her/him support by disclosing her/his condition. However, a person is not obliged to disclose his or her status. Positive living means that one is aware that people living with HIV are often discriminated against and she/he is ready to face and challenge such rejections without allowing these prejudices to affect her/him emotionally and spiritually.

Positive living with HIV means maintaining good personal hygiene, eating a healthy diet, taking medication as prescribed and completing the course of treatment, exercising regularly, getting enough rest and relaxation, get medical care when ill or if you see any signs of infection, practicing safer sex at all times. Positive living means getting emotional help if you realise you are not coping with your emotions as well as you would like to, thinking positively knowing that you can live with the virus for many years.

Conclude by reading "Remember 7.1"

Session 19: What cancers can affect the reproductive system of females and males?

Allow the participants to give their own views and write the on a flip chart. Go through the presentations and identify issues that need to be clarified and explain in details. In details go though the following cancers that affect the reproductive system: Cervical cancer (including the human papillomavirus), Breast Cancer (include breast self-examination) and testicular cancer (include testicular self-examination).

Exercise 10: What is gender?

Ask participants to do Exercise 10 from the "Get to know yourself: A sexual health guide for young people" book. Allow participants to give their own views about what the facilitator asked her participants and write the on a flip chart and leave them for discussion later. Then ask participants to answer discuss the questions in Exercise 10 and present their views at plenary.

Activity 31

Hand out a list of gender statements to all participants. In groups ask them to identify statements that are gender and those that are sex. Go through the statements to check if they have identified them properly and correct where necessary.

Activity 32

What is gender based violence?
Allow participants to discuss in groups and report to plenary. Go through their presentations to add and correct where necessary.

Activity 33

Ask participants to discuss in their groups the following questions:

- What is my role and responsibility in promoting gender equality among my peers and community?
- What can I do to help someone who is being abused or has been abused (sexually, physically or emotionally)?

Allow the participants to present their views and discuss in plenary.

Conclude by reading "Remember: 8.1" from the "Get to know yourself: A sexual health guide for young people" book.

Session 21: What is my role and responsibility as a young person in my community?

Activity 34

In groups, ask participants to discuss their roles and responsibilities by answering the following questions:

- What is my role and responsibility to me?
- What is my role and responsibility to my home and family?
- What is my role and responsibility to my friends?
- What is my role and responsibility to my community?
- What is my role and responsibility to my school or workplace?
- What is my role and responsibility to my country?
- What is my role and responsibility to the world?
- What steps am I going to take to be or remain physically, spiritually and socially healthy?
- What steps am I going to take to make my family live a healthy fulfilling life?
- What steps am I going to take to make sure that my community is healthy?
- What steps am I going to take to ensure that the knowledge and skill that I have gained during this workshop is disseminated or benefits my family and community?

Allow participants to discuss their answers and discuss. Summarise the presentations. Conclude by reading the "I am sexually health" poem from the "Get to know yourself: A sexual health guide for young people" book

Session 22: Summary of the day and workshop

Evaluation of the day

To evaluate the day put the following on a flip chart: "What have I learnt?" "What have I unlearned?" "The message I am taking with me" Ask each participant to give an answer for each question and statement. Write their answers on a flip chart. Paste it on the wall.

Summary of the workshop

Summarise by revisiting the expectations, fears, aims and objectives of the workshop and discuss with the participants on whether they have been met or not. Then ask them to list individually two things from the workshop that were important and of benefit to them.

Thank them heartily and formally close the workshop.

Session 23: Evaluation and closure

Invite the participants to complete the evaluation form before they leave. Thank them again.

LET THE SEXUAL HEALTH CANDLE GIVE LIGHT TO HEALTHY LIVING AMONG YOUNG PEOPLE IN THE COMMUNITY!